Science Fiction and the Ethics of Artificial Wombs

Reproductive Ethics: Critical Perspectives

Series editors: Rebecca Bennett (University of Manchester, UK) and Panagiota Nakou (University of Nicosia Medical School, Cyprus)

This series explores, illuminates and ignites debates in the growing field of reproductive ethics. At a time when ethical questions surrounding reproduction have never been more in the spotlight, *Reproductive Ethics: Critical Perspectives* investigates ethical issues around emerging technologies, reproductive choice, reproductive justice and the scope of legitimate interests of the state in reproductive decisions. Bringing together scholars from a number of disciplines including ethics, philosophy, law, sociology and feminist thought, this series provides a reliable source of authoritative books that tackle timely and pressing issues, from prenatal screening for disabilities to the overturning of Roe v. Wade. Topics of interest include, but are no means limited to:

- Partial or full artificial wombs (ectogenesis)
- The possibility of uterine transplants
- Surrogacy markets
- Proposed screening for substance/alcohol use in pregnancy
- Childbirth
- Disparities in maternal healthcare
- Pro-natalism
- Pre-implantation and pre-natal screening
- Whole genome screening
- IVF and artificial reproductive technology
- Abortion and access to terminations
- Men's reproductive rights and male pregnancy
- Transgender reproductive autonomy
- Forced sterilization
- Contraception
- Regulation and policy to encourage an increase in birth rates
- Reproductive coercion in marginalized communities
- Environmental factors affecting fertility

Science Fiction and the Ethics of Artificial Wombs

Reproductive Futures

Evie Kendal

BLOOMSBURY ACADEMIC
LONDON • NEW YORK • OXFORD • NEW DELHI • SYDNEY

BLOOMSBURY ACADEMIC
Bloomsbury Publishing Plc, 50 Bedford Square, London, WC1B 3DP, UK
Bloomsbury Publishing Inc, 1359 Broadway, New York, NY 10018, USA
Bloomsbury Publishing Ireland, 29 Earlsfort Terrace, Dublin 2, D02 AY28, Ireland

First published in Great Britain 2026

Series design by Jade Barnett
Cover image: koto_feja / Getty Images

A catalogue record for this book is available from the British Library.

A catalog record for this book is available from the Library of Congress.

ISBN: HB: 978-1-3505-4297-6
ePDF: 978-1-3505-4298-3
eBook: 978-1-3505-4299-0

Series: Reproductive Ethics: Critical Perspectives

Typeset by Newgen KnowledgeWorks Pvt. Ltd., Chennai, India

For product safety related questions contact productsafety@bloomsbury.com.

Contents

Acknowledgements vi

Introduction 1

1. Locating ectogenesis 15
2. The role of imagination in bioethics 45
3. Science fiction engaging with bioethics 69
4. Bioethics engaging with science fiction 93
5. Things to do with (science fiction) stories 119

Conclusion 157

Notes 163
Bibliography 203
Index 229

Acknowledgements

Thanks are due to many people for sharing their insights into the issues discussed in this book. Of note are Dr Ben Beccari, Dr M. L. Pitone, Ms Alexandra Stokes, Dr Gabriel Garcia-Ochoa and all the members of the Sídhe Feminist Literary Collective for providing specific comments and advice. Acknowledgements also to Professor Emeritus Andrew Milner and Professors Catherine Mills, Olivia Khoo, Justin Oakley and Basia Diug for supervising the doctoral project that provided the starting point for this book many years ago. Thanks also to the staff at the Merrill Collection of Science Fiction, Speculation and Fantasy at the Toronto Public Library for providing access to various special editions of the science fiction texts considered here and the Yale Interdisciplinary Center for Bioethics for facilitating access to their library of bioethics texts and the Beinecke Rare Book and Manuscript Library. Thanks are also due to the Berggruen Institute for commissioning a related fictional work as part of the Life, Otherwise exhibition. A final thanks to the anonymous peer reviewers for their detailed and constructive feedback.

Funding to produce or present the research contained herein has been provided by the Australian Government Department of Education; the Brocher Foundation Visiting Scholars' Residency program; the Japanese Association of Bioethics-International Association of Bioethics (JAB-IAB) Fellowship; Monash University (including the Monash-Warwick Alliance); Deakin University's Science and Society Network (SSN); the Korean Society for Transplantation (ATW Secretariat); the Transplantation Society of Australia and New Zealand (TSANZ); the Queensland Government Department of Tourism, Innovation and Sport; TEDxRoma; Chamber Made; the Cécile Parrish Memorial Fund; and the Julia Peluso Memorial Prize. This book was written under the employment of Swinburne University of Technology in Victoria, Australia, and supported by the School of Health Sciences, Department of Biomedical, Health and Exercise Sciences and the Iverson Health Innovation Research Institute.

Introduction

Since at least the 1950s, the possibility of growing a human foetus outside of the organic womb has fascinated scientists and fiction authors alike.[1] Whether it be full ectogenesis,[2] for example, growing a foetus externally from conception, or partial ectogenesis, an extension of current artificial incubation methods used in neonatal care, such technology carries many ethical considerations. It is therefore not surprising that the issues surrounding whether we should allow the development of artificial wombs, and if so, for what purposes, are hotly debated in bioethics literature. As a technology that is still largely speculative, ectogenesis can be found in several science-fictional texts focused on exploring possible futures, and references to these texts frequently turn up in bioethical debate. But what attitudes and beliefs might such visions of the future of reproductive medicine expose in the real world? This book seeks to explore this question, with particular reference to science fiction film and literature.

This introduction will briefly consider how public perceptions of reproductive biotechnologies can promote or frustrate various agendas connected with ectogenesis, before considering how pronatalist beliefs contribute to societal views of the role of women in human reproduction. Core arguments will be placed within the context of the existing scholarly literature on ectogenesis and science fiction in bioethics. Overall, the aim throughout this book is to explore how the benefits of ectogenesis for promoting sexual equality can be better represented in narratives from within bioethics, science fiction and, especially, bioethics scholarship that engages with science fiction. By considering how and why representations of emerging technologies matter, this book will develop a methodology for more effectively integrating stories of speculative technologies into ethical debate.

Why perceptions of reproductive biotechnologies really matter

Among the advantages ectogenesis could contribute to society are improved health for women,[3] through avoiding the physical and emotional toll of pregnancy and childbirth; greater reproductive autonomy for parents who either cannot or do not wish to be pregnant (including the socially infertile); improved health for foetuses through enhanced control over foetal development, nutrition and the avoidance of teratogens; and the opportunity to save foetuses born prematurely, or otherwise destined for termination. In her article, 'Not of Woman Born', Jennifer S. Hendricks says bioethicists and legal commentators generally summarize such arguments as 'better for women, better than surrogacy, better for babies, and better than abortion'.[4] For women, the considerable discomfort associated with pregnancy-related illnesses, such as morning sickness, coupled with the pain and suffering associated with childbirth itself, justifies exploring alternatives to physical gestation for prospective mothers and surrogates. There is also the potential suffering women face if they have difficulty conceiving or sustaining a pregnancy, or are infertile, both of which can cause physical and psychological pain associated with pregnancy, even when no pregnancy occurs. Recognizing that in addition to these typical burdens, up to fifteen per cent of pregnant women develop potentially life-threatening complications associated with pregnancy, the possibility to procreate without these risks is likely to appeal to some.[5] In her book, *Full Surrogacy Now: Feminism Against Family*, Sophie Lewis writes:

> It is a wonder we let fetuses inside of us. Unlike almost all other animals, hundreds of thousands of humans die because of their pregnancies every year … This situation is social, not simply 'natural'. Things are like this for political and economic reasons: we *made* them this way.
>
> Pregnancy undoubtedly has its pleasures; natality is unique. That is why, even as others suffer deeply from their coerced participation in pregnancy, many people excluded from the experience for whatever reason – be they cis, trans, or nonbinary – feel deeply bereft. But even so, and even in full recognition of the sense of the sublime that people experience in gestating, it is remarkable that there isn't more consistent support for research into alleviating the *problem* of pregnancy.[6]

While maternal morbidity and mortality certainly constitute a significant part of the problem at stake here, the fact that there are currently no alternatives to biological gestation goes further than just risking the health and safety of specific women – it represents a lack of choice for all prospective parents. A woman may wish to avoid accepting the hazards of pregnancy for herself, just as any partner/s she has may wish to avoid imposing them on her for their joint reproductive endeavour. Likewise, while the socio-economic and political disadvantages Lewis refers to can (and should) be addressed as social, rather than biological, phenomena, it will always remain the case that some people simply cannot, or do not *wish* to, gestate. It is particularly in this space that reproductive biotechnologies, including ectogenesis, would continue to meet specific needs for women in family creation projects.

Additional potential benefits of ectogenesis include the ability to cater to the needs of gay male couples and single men who wish to procreate without engaging a surrogate, or women who suffer from absolute uterine factor infertility, for which no alternative fertility treatments are effective except in the rare case where a transplant uterus is available and there are no contraindications for transplantation.[7] Uterine transplants are still in clinical trials in several countries, with increasing numbers of successful live births being achieved.[8] Even so, it is unclear whether this intervention will be offered to transgender women in the future, suggesting ectogenesis might remain an important option for these women in particular.[9] In the future, it is even possible that bioengineered wombs might have a role to play in both ectogenesis and transplant medicine.[10] With regard to promoting foetal interests, the opportunity to gestate a foetus with no threat of accidental or intentional exposure to harmful substances can also be viewed as a desirable possibility. Yashita Khulbe et al. also note that from a public health perspective, a cost-effective artificial womb could prevent various developmental issues associated with infections, intrauterine growth retardation, placental insufficiency, prematurity, and birth injuries, at the population level.[11] Zhelan Huang et al. add to this list the possible protective role of an artificial womb against the high risk of intercranial haemorrhage, limb adhesion and malformation, nutrition-related complications (including necrotizing enterocolitis), hypothermia and dehydration frequently impacting extremely premature infants kept in standard air-based incubators.[12] However, despite this broad potential for appeal, perceptions of ectogenesis, particularly among conservatives, currently pose an obstacle to research in the area.

A qualitative study conducted in Israel by Frida Simonstein and Michal Mashiach-Eizenberg illustrates that the proposed uses of ectogenesis influence whether the technology is considered acceptable. When ectogenesis was proposed as a method of saving foetuses, respondents viewed it favourably, but when suggested as a method of alleviating the burdens of reproduction for women, it was opposed. These authors note that while pregnancy 'can be deadly', the lack of concern over women's welfare in pregnancy is likely because 'reproductive hazards have traditionally been viewed as women's fate and, therefore, taken for granted'.[13] This is precisely where science fiction can contribute to the bioethical debate on ectogenesis, as in fiction's realm of suspended disbelief what is taken for granted in our everyday reality is subject to radical destabilization. As Anna Smajdor asserts, the 'necessity of women for gestating and nurturing society's children is so entrenched in our consciousness that we fail to recognize that we could change the situation'.[14] This poverty of imagination[15] may be understandable in a world that has never seen an alternative method of gestation in action, but in the imaginary worlds of science fiction, there is an opportunity to explore what human society might look like were childbearing no longer necessarily linked to women's bodies. Thus, when it comes to perceptions of ectogenesis, science fiction provides many visions of possible future uses that might impact how artificial gestation is imagined.

A poverty of imagination

One cause of the lack of imagination when it comes to reproductive futures is the pervasive influence of pronatalism on understandings of women's roles in society. Pronatalism is a belief system that promotes childbearing, often through manufacturing a romanticized view of parenthood and perceived social duty to reproduce.[16] Diana Meyers claims that pronatalist dogma seeks to perpetuate the idea that motherhood is 'inevitable' for women, thereby preventing many from seriously contemplating a future without children.[17] While pronatalism exerts pressure on people of all genders to reproduce, the physiological differences between typical male and female experiences of human reproduction are fairly obvious: women get pregnant, whereas men do not. Thus, the burdens associated with pregnancy – physically, socially and economically – are disproportionately borne by women. Ectogenesis has the potential to undermine any assumption that such an unequal division of reproductive labour across the sexes is inevitable, facilitating a future in which men and women contribute more equally to procreation. While the risks associated with the extraction of sperm and ova can never be wholly equivalent, allowing for an alternative to the more burdensome element of gestation for women represents a significant step towards equalizing male and female contributions to human reproduction.[18] But achieving sexual equality is a utopian impulse, and supporting ectogenesis research on these grounds requires an ability to imagine a future free from the patriarchal values that assign certain positions to women in society and perpetuate myths about motherhood.

The benefits of achieving greater sexual equality in reproduction extend beyond family-making and parenting roles. Rosemarie Tong claims that the 'joy of giving birth – invoked so frequently in this society – is a patriarchal myth', designed to keep women in the home.[19] She notes that were ectogenesis an alternative to physical gestation, the 'primary rationale' for restricting women's access to public life would disappear, thus promoting a more equal distribution of social benefits in the future.[20] However, one does not have to believe reproduction is the 'primary' cause of sexual inequality to understand it is nevertheless a significant contributor. Ectogenesis may also be viewed as a *necessary* option to improve this situation without being a *sufficient* one – in fact, without a commitment to other social changes aimed at improving women's equality, emerging reproductive technologies could rather exacerbate existing inequalities. This was the focus of the predecessor to this text, published in 2015 before the breakthroughs in bio-bag research rekindled interest in the topic of ectogenesis in mainstream bioethics scholarship, as will be discussed in Chapter 1.[21] Even respecting the above constraints, providing an alternative site for gestation inherently challenges many assumptions that perpetuate women's disadvantage in society.

Embracing the potential for ectogenesis to contribute to women's empowerment would likely also require that new narratives be created around it to counteract the effect of the culturally entrenched myths about women and motherhood that pronatalism espouses. Linking the concept of ectogenesis to Donna Haraway's *A Cyborg Manifesto* (1984), Dion Farquhar claims:

> Opponents of ectogenesis cannot imagine other non(counter)canonical, discursive, or textual appropriations, allegorical rewritings, unintended consequences, or liberatory possibilities that cyborgian ectogenesis might come to offer some women.[22]

As in the case of Haraway's cyborg, a positive counter-narrative for ectogenesis relies on a breakdown of traditional boundaries concerning gender and sexuality in society. This has the potential to benefit not only women but also men and non-binary prospective parents as well.

As one of the primary spaces in which we imagine possible futures, science fiction contains many useful discussions of alternative social realities. As Dennis

Livingston notes, science fiction provides a 'laboratory' for the imagination, a space to explore radical alternatives to our lived experience.[23] Canonical science fiction author Ursula K. Le Guin describes futuristic science fiction in a similar way in an interview for *Smithsonian* magazine, when she notes: 'The future is a safe, sterile laboratory for trying out ideas in … a means of thinking about reality, a method'.[24] However, there is currently a lack of imagination evidenced in much of the science fiction depicting ectogenesis, particularly regarding its potential to promote sexual equality in human reproduction. Here, imagination may refer to the manipulation of mental images, consideration of counterfactual scenarios or simulation of another's experiences or situation.[25] As such, imagination is important for considering the world not as it is, but as it could be.

This element of experimentation goes some way towards explaining why speculative fictions can be useful for normative ethics. However, Amy Mullin argues that 'acts of imagining and failures to imagine can both be morally significant. Failures to imagine are perhaps most obviously morally culpable.'[26] A poverty of imagination within the science fiction genre regarding the potential for ectogenesis to promote sexual equality thus becomes an ethical issue worthy of consideration. When the source material within the genre is overwhelmingly negative, as will be argued throughout this book, its use in bioethical debate is likely to follow suit. Mullin continues by claiming that while it might be inappropriate to hold a single fictional work responsible for 'preventing us from imagining situations and events in morally relevant ways', a genre may be a more valid target for such accusations, as readers may develop habits from repeated exposure to generic tropes.[27]

The relevant habits here include the negative reactions inspired by the oft-grotesque renderings of artificial gestation in science fiction. While this situation may well be problematic in its own right, it is the over-reliance in bioethics scholarship on negative representations of ectogenesis from science fiction that is the central concern here. In this, a 'failure to imagine' is being exploited for rhetorical gain to promote a techno-conservative view of human reproduction and definitions of family. This also highlights how the tools of literary analysis, such as narratology, can contribute to debate in this area, with its primary focus not on the interpretation of individual texts but rather on the broader structural elements of texts and genres. Positive representations of ectogenesis do exist in science fiction; however, these are in the minority and are almost entirely ignored in bioethics scholarship, despite the frequency with which the negative depictions are utilized. Both these choices carry ethical significance and suggest that a more balanced use of 'bioethics-in-literature' methodologies could be pursued, which resist the impetus to reduce works of fiction into simplified moral principles or rely solely on their potential shock value in bioethical debate.

The history of bioethics scholarship on ectogenesis and science fiction

Placing the arguments in this book within the wider bioethics scholarship first requires an investigation of the historical literature on ectogenesis and the role of science fiction in bioethical debate. There is a considerable body of work on the ethics of ectogenesis, with particular concentrations seen around the 1970s, surrounding the advent of *in vitro* fertilization (IVF) in 1978, and the early 2000s, following the first successful animal experiments using artificial wombs in the mid-1990s.[28] There are also several influential works focused on the role of science fiction in bioethics and the 'bioethics-in-literature' field. One of the earliest and still one of the most influential texts supporting the development of ectogenesis to promote greater sexual equality in reproduction is Shulamith Firestone's 1970s radical feminist manifesto, *The Dialectic of Sex*.[29] In this text, Firestone argues that women's oppression stems from their biological capacity for childbearing, and thus alternative methods for propagating the human species, such as ectogenesis, must be developed. What separates Firestone's vision from many that followed it is that she argued for the total abolition of biological pregnancy as a necessary step towards sexual equality, rather than promoting ectogenesis as an option for those women who would choose it. In this way, the experience of pregnancy is only considered at the community level. Almost twenty years later, Julien Murphy's article 'Is Pregnancy Necessary?' similarly questions whether women should 'as a group, be liberated from the responsibility of child-bearing?'[30] Considering Firestone's argument that reproduction should cease to be viewed as 'women's work', Murphy outlines a number of arguments for and against ectogenesis that apply the potential pros and cons of the technology to women as a marginalized group.[31] Firestone imagines a future revolution that can benefit all women, including through the development of alternatives to physical gestation, whereas Murphy remains concerned that as a group women might ultimately be worse off should ectogenesis be developed. Nevertheless, she notes most opposing arguments fail to hold up under scrutiny, including claims that ectogenesis will inevitably lead to the exploitation or devaluing of women as a group.[32] In her 'History of Gestation Outside the Body', Claire Horn claims Firestone is 'often misrepresented as an enthusiastic technopositivist who uncritically embraced ectogenesis' but reminds readers that *The Dialectic of Sex* also contains Firestone's warning that 'in the hands of current scientists, few of whom are feminist or even female', the technology could not be trusted.[33] Elsewhere, Horn argues that beliefs that the biological disentanglement of gestation from women's bodies will succeed in 'de-gendering' gestation are misguided, as she suggests it is the law that needs to change for this to occur, not biology.[34] Nevertheless, it remains the case that whatever else is required for it to be successful, Firestone's proposed revolution is entirely dependent on alternatives to biological gestation being developed.

For the opposing radical feminist stance, Gena Corea's *The Mother Machine* explores the 'brothel' and 'farming' models of social control over women, arguing that artificial gestation may represent a fundamental harm to women's social power as a group, as the patriarchal authority will no longer need to invest in husbanding (or 'farming') women to obtain offspring (crops). Corea argues that taking away women's fundamental role as the creators of human life will leave them no use in a patriarchal society beyond sex work.[35] This idea features in several of the dystopian narratives discussed in this book but is one of the more sensational arguments against ectogenesis. Other feminist authors opposed to the expansion of reproductive technologies include Barbara Katz Rothman, Robyn Rowland and Andrea Dworkin, whose arguments are similarly concerned with the potential for these technologies to be co-opted to serve patriarchal objectives. Rothman's book, *A Bun in the Oven*, describes an alleged shift away from unique birthing experiences in society, such as home-births, in favour of an over-medicalized, hospital-based 'industrial birth' system, in which women's embodied experiences of pregnancy and childbirth are largely ignored.[36] She suggests that increased technological interference in pregnancy and childbirth has had a negative impact on women's health and safety, a view shared by Rowland and Dworkin, who further claim that it is men who control these technologies, often to the detriment of the women who wish to use them.[37] These three authors and Corea all argue that artificial wombs pose a threat to women's social status, as they would replace the need for women to gestate the next generation.[38] At the same time, Jan Zimmerman argued of ectogenesis:

> While such technologies may offer women freedom from childbearing, which has been a form of female bondage, they also offer men an unprecedented opportunity to assert control over the one aspect of the life process which has eluded them until now. … Men have a long record of usurping control of medical technologies.[39]

It is further suggested that women would be unable to stop the development of such technologies, but it is recommended that as a group they 'park themselves in the path of technological determinism' and focus on influencing how such technologies would be applied in society.[40]

In many cases, the above arguments fall into what Farquhar calls 'fundamentalist feminist discourse', as they consider women's experiences of pregnancy and motherhood as universal, with no allowances for differences of race or class.[41] Such perspectives are most likely to take an all-or-nothing stance toward reproductive technologies – whether that be Firestone's enthusiasm for eradicating biological gestation or Rowland's general opposition to IVF and related technologies. Mary Anne Case's definition of feminist fundamentalism is also fitting here, as she claims it entails being 'deeply and profoundly committed to the equality of the sexes', adding that for her personally, such a commitment represents 'my fundament, my root, my base'.[42] While some people adopt the term to refer to people who self-identify as feminist from within a fundamentalist faith tradition, Case notes that 'the hallmark of fundamentalism is an unwillingness to compromise' and differentiates this from perfectionism, which she claims is a 'willingness to impose on others … perfectionism speaks in the second or third person – it is about what "you" or "they" should or must do'.[43] Wholesale rejection of either biological gestation or the use of reproductive biotechnologies due to concerns about patriarchal appropriation treats women and their experiences of reproduction in the aggregate, a collective of potentially pregnant persons, rather than individuals likely to have vastly different views on what procreation should look like.

Contrasting the above group-focused perspectives, works by Peter Singer and Deane Wells focus on individual rights to pursue ectogenesis, irrespective of any communal attitude toward the technology.[44] They summarize their argument as follows:

> Women would not, after all, be compelled to use the new method; all it would do is provide them with a new option. If they wished to avoid pregnancy and childbirth while still having a child of their own, they could; if they preferred the traditional experience, they could of course go through with it all in the traditional manner. … It is not necessary for us to take sides on this issue, however, because women are responsible agents capable of choosing for themselves whether to have the experience in question. It would be an act of extraordinary paternalism – never mind about male chauvinism – for a [predominantly male] government to tell women that because it knew that pregnancy was good for them, it would not allow the development of alternative means of producing babies. … The most

> likely situation, in fact, is that ectogenesis, like most technologies, will suit some women and not others. The fact that it will not suit everyone is no reason why those women who prefer it should not have access to it.[45]

This argument fits well with the liberal feminist perspective adopted in this book, as it focuses on individual freedoms, rather than community values. Similarly, Smajdor's controversial 2007 article, 'The Moral Imperative for Ectogenesis', and its 2012 follow-up, 'In Defense of Ectogenesis', approach this issue from the perspective of promoting individual choice.[46] Comparing the experience of procreation between men and women, Smajdor claims '[t]he choices and risks open to them are vastly unequal', such that even if an individual woman voluntarily chooses to take on the risks of pregnancy, she is still disadvantaged relative to a man who wishes to procreate, for whom such risks are never a factor.[47] The right of individual women to choose less risky methods of reproducing, should they personally desire this, forms the basis of Smajdor's support for ectogenesis.

According to Brenda Russell, Debra Oswald and MaryKate Cotter, liberal feminism 'advocates for achieving gender equality through political and legal reforms, aiming to establish equal rights and opportunities for both men and women'.[48] As such, it looks for laws and policies that treat men and women differently and tries to remedy this, rather than radically opposing the underlying social structures that have led to this inequality, including capitalism. Thus, Clare Chambers notes that liberal feminism is sometimes described as being 'just about equality', conceptualizing 'freedom primarily in terms of choice'.[49] This aligns with liberalism more broadly, with its focus on promoting individual freedom, which Amy R. Baehr notes can either be defined as 'freedom from coercive interference' or 'freedom as personal autonomy – living a life of one's own choosing'.[50] However, as with all areas of bioethics, demonstrating genuine freedom of choice and informed consent in reproduction is complicated. Promoting the principle of autonomy, as the cornerstone of much of Western medical ethics, often assumes free and informed decision-making is equally possible (and desirable) for everyone once overt barriers and forms of coercion are removed. Julinna C. Oxley claims that as the 'oldest version of feminism', liberal feminism has accumulated much criticism over time, including for 'overlook[ing] differences of race, socioeconomic status, and sexual orientation relevant to an accurate assessment of women's situation'.[51] This criticism not only highlights that some laws and policies disproportionately impact some women over others but also that just removing legal barriers to gender equality is insufficient in cases where there are intersectional issues at play. Nevertheless, both liberalism, in general, and liberal feminism, more specifically, can be applied to defend women's freedom to choose if and how to pursue the goal of family creation and to the legal systems needed to support procreative liberty and women's empowerment.

The position taken in this book most closely aligns to the individual liberty perspective of liberal feminism but is sympathetic to many of the concerns Firestone notes regarding the inescapable inequality of biological reproduction. The fundamentalist feminist perspectives that attempt to universalize women's experiences of reproduction are less suitable for the highly individualized nature of reproductive medicine as it is currently practiced in Western society, and thus are not considered in any detail. However, it is recognized that these arguments are likely to carry much more weight among societies arranged along more communitarian values.

With regard to the use of science fiction in bioethical discussions of reproductive biotechnologies, Susan M. Squier's 1994 book *Babies in Bottles*, provides a useful starting point.[52] Squier recognizes the unique relationship between fiction and science, illustrating how the representation of new reproductive biotechnologies impacts public reactions to these scientific advancements. Sherryl Vint's edited collection, 'Science Fiction and Biopolitics', explores Squier's analysis, claiming her argument is too pessimistic regarding the impact of science fiction on public debate.[53] The stance adopted here agrees with Vint that there is a role for science fiction to play in shaping the future, not just prefiguring it. Science fiction has the potential to contribute meaningfully to bioethical debate focused on emerging technologies, but this requires an understanding of the relationship between bioethics and the imagination, and, in turn, the imagination and science fiction. In terms of promoting sexual equality in reproduction, realizing this potential requires careful consideration of the use and impact of science-fictional references in bioethical debate.

Historical perspectives on ectogenesis ethics still influence current bioethics scholarship, as will be considered in detail in Chapter 1. What this book adds to the overall body of literature on this topic is an exploration of how the use of science fiction in bioethics scholarship could be improved in the future through applying tools of literary analysis to the texts being invoked, especially drawing on the field of narratology. Furthermore, it addresses the role of imagination and storytelling in bioethics, illustrating that science-fictional references can serve a valuable function in communicating bioethical arguments.

Aims and outline

This book explores the current and future role of science fiction in bioethical debates surrounding ectogenesis, in the light of the fundamental contribution this technology could make to promoting sexual equality in human reproduction. It begins by exploring the potential benefits of ectogenesis, especially for women, with particular focus on the possibility of avoiding the risks and burdens of biological pregnancy. Such benefits also include providing a means to gestate offspring for prospective parents who lack a functional womb, such as women who are born without a uterus or lose theirs to injury or cancer, and gay male couples and single men who cannot or do not wish to engage a surrogate. It then continues by examining how these various benefits are deprioritised or ignored in many science-fictional texts depicting the technology. A detailed description of the artificial womb as a trope in science fiction is included, alongside an analysis of the frequent association of this future reproductive technology with other scientific and medical developments, such as cloning and human augmentation. The use of science fiction in bioethical debates surrounding ectogenesis is then explored, concluding that the dominant purpose of science-fictional references and images in bioethics scholarship is to establish a link between this technology and a variety of negative social and political outcomes. Throughout this book, it is argued that the fictional representations of ectogenesis referenced in bioethics scholarship are often sensationalist and misleading, perpetuating various stereotypes about gender roles in procreation and promoting the idea that ectogenesis will inevitably lead to catastrophe. The final section proposes alternative ways of engaging with science fiction in bioethical debate, such that it can reach its potential as a means of communicating biotechnological knowledge and exploring speculative futures, rather than being used to prejudice others against a technology that could benefit the lives of women and prospective parents.

This book aims to expose the ethical implications and opportunities arising from the relationship between bioethics and the science fiction genre. Exploring who is using science-fictional references to discuss reproductive technologies, and to what end, will assist in establishing why it is important to understand the potential impact of representation on the bioethical debate surrounding ectogenesis. While the technology appears in various science fiction texts, especially those within the utopian and dystopian fiction sub-genre, positive feminist utopias incorporating ectogenesis are under-represented in both science fiction as a genre and the bioethics literature that engages with it. Furthermore, while there are many reasons for developing ectogenesis provided in science-fictional texts, the potential for achieving sexual equality is rarely the primary motivation and, in many cases, is not considered at all. Instead, the continual association in science-fictional texts of artificial gestation with other allegedly sinister goals, such as human reproductive cloning and genetic engineering, often conflates concerns regarding ectogenesis with other biotechnologies and political agendas. Such a misrepresentation of what ectogenesis necessarily entails serves to obscure how it might function beneficially within the suite of assisted reproductive technologies already available.

Due to their inherently speculative nature, science fiction, and particularly dystopian narratives, are powerful persuasive tools shaping how we imagine and pursue possible futures.[54] As such, there is a need to apply a feminist critique to the representation of ectogenesis in science fiction to explore the apparent lack of vision regarding the potential for this technology to promote greater sexual equality in human reproduction. Critically examining the socio-political motivations behind invoking science fiction in bioethical debate makes apparent the importance of representation on how science and technology are integrated into society. This examination will consider the role of moral intuition and the influence of the 'yuck factor' in bioethical debates, as these both demonstrate how perceptions can be influenced through rhetoric and imagery drawn from fictional texts.

1

Locating ectogenesis

Before any claim can be made about the potential use and misuse of science fiction in bioethical debates regarding ectogenesis, it is first necessary to establish the problems this emerging technology could help solve. This chapter explores these alongside the ethical arguments in favour of ectogenesis that justify the development of this technology.

The idea of artificial gestation inspires strong feelings in many people. Leslie Cannold's research on women's attitudes towards ectogenesis, published in 1995, indicated that even in cases where women were strongly opposed to abortion, they did not consider ectogenesis a desirable alternative to termination for an unwanted pregnancy.[1] Her qualitative study merely posited ectogenesis as an alternative to abortion, rather than as an alternative to biological gestation in general, so responses were often focused on a perceived abandonment of maternal responsibility if transferring a foetus to an artificial womb for subsequent adoption. The bioethicists to be discussed in this chapter, however, have focused on various other potential uses for the technology, including catering to a woman's desire to reproduce without pregnancy.

This chapter also provides a brief overview of the state of the science of ectogenesis research before exploring in more detail the issues of sexual inequality in human reproduction that this technology could help address. This is important context when considering why using negative representations of the technology might be ethically suspect, given the significant risks and burdens of reproduction ectogenesis could alleviate for women.

Ectogenesis: The state of the science

The need to consider the potential future impact of ectogenesis on society stems in part from recent developments in various 'precursor' technologies, such as miniaturized oxygenators that may in the future serve as part of an artificial placenta.[2] One of the more recent forays into artificial gestation was conducted in 2016 by Emily A. Partridge et al.'s team at the Children's Hospital of Philadelphia Research Institute, in which premature lamb foetuses were successfully incubated for several weeks in a newly developed 'bio-bag'.[3] This system involves a sealed plastic bag filled with an electrolyte solution similar to amniotic fluid and a pumpless arteriovenous oxygenator circuit that allows constant fluid exchange.[4] In a news article for *Nature* in September 2023, Max Kozlov noted these scientists were seeking approval to begin human trials of their Extra-Uterine Environment for Newborn Development (EXTEND) system.[5] A meeting of the US Food and Drug Administration (FDA) was scheduled that month to discuss the proposal,[6] but limited the focus of that discussion to potential uses for treating premature infants (around twenty-two to twenty-four weeks' gestation).[7] A similar system was also developed in Perth, Australia, in 2017, representing a collaboration between the Women's and Infant's Research Foundation and Tohoku University in Japan.[8] This platform, known as the Ex-Vivo Uterine Environment (EVE), was also successfully trialled using premature lamb foetuses.[9] In both cases, researchers have made it clear that they are not pursuing full ectogenesis but rather hope to enhance the survival rates of infants born prematurely.

While such ectogenesis experiments are showing promising results in animal studies, up until this point, oxygenation has represented the major obstacle to achieving artificial gestation in humans. It is telling that one of the scientists involved in the bio-bag project responded to queries about human testing by stating: 'It's complete science fiction to think that you can take an embryo and get it through the early developmental process and put it on our machine without the mother being the critical element there.'[10] Nevertheless, once a viable method of providing oxygen and nutrients to the foetus is established, scientists working in the field generally agree that the other technical requirements for human ectogenesis should be relatively easy to meet. These include the need to create a three-dimensional 'shell' to provide a site for embryo implantation[11] and to develop an artificial substitute for amniotic fluid.[12] Regarding the first requirement, experimental chambers have already been developed using explanted uterine tissue, synthetic materials (like the bio-bag models) and endometrial cells grown on biodegradable scaffolding.[13] As for the second, synthetic amniotic fluid has already been successfully trialled in animal experiments.[14] In late 2023, Braxton Forde et al. also trialled a synthetic amniotic fluid called 'Amnio-well', which they claimed mimicked the composition of its human counterpart in terms of electrolyte, pH, albumin and glucose concentration. These authors reported 'normalization of cellular signalling and less cell death' in the cultured amniotic epithelial cells exposed to Amnio-well compared to the sample exposed to the standard amnioinfusion preparation used before foetal interventions.[15]

Perhaps most significantly, in 2019, a grant was awarded to researchers at Eindhoven University of Technology in the Netherlands to develop the first prototype artificial womb to help incubate prematurely born human infants, which is anticipated to build on the bio-bag concept.[16] A recent doctoral project at this institution by Juliette van Haren focused on developing safe foetal transfer methods from the organic to artificial womb. According to a summary of her work, this would involve 'a wound spreader, coupling elements and a biobag filled with amniotic fluid', in other words, the creation of a fluid-filled portal where the foetus would travel from one gestational site to the other without being exposed to the outside world.[17] This is significant, as lung underdevelopment is the main cause of morbidity and mortality among premature infants, and maintaining a foetus in a fluid-filled environment would prevent the transition from foetal to neonatal physiology that necessitates the ability to breathe oxygen from the external environment.[18] As such, it would allow the foetal lungs to continue normal maturation, thereby increasing survival odds.[19] This team also published a study in 2023 investigating the views of medical specialists with expertise in vessel cannulation to discuss the plausibility of establishing a 'connection between the infant's native umbilical cord and an artificial placenta system through cannulation', finding various points of consensus across participants regarding a preferred technique to achieve this goal.[20] Beyond the benefit of avoiding cases of extreme prematurity leading to lung failure, Felix De Bie et al. claim that partial ectogenesis could also be used to 'improve the feasibility and safety of targeted, repeated prenatal therapy (fetal surgery, pharmaco-, gene or stem cell therapy)', with possible, but as yet unconfirmed, benefits to the pregnant women of these cases.[21] While the scope of such use cases will remain unknown for some time, neonatologists generally agree that delaying the need for conventional positive pressure ventilation will prevent lung damage in premature infants and improve survivability.[22]

As far back as the 1990s, Nobuya Unno et al. suggested that fluid-based incubators would be more effective than the current air-based humidicrib models used in neonatal intensive care units; however, as noted above, such systems are still not available for human infants.[23] Nevertheless, trials of partial ectogenesis are continuing around the world using different species at different gestational ages. One particularly interesting case was a species preservation project in Australia in 2009, which artificially incubated late-stage wobbegong shark embryos in an acrylic tank until independent viability.[24] This latter example also served as a cautionary tale for others working in artificial gestation at the time, after a public outcry regarding the possibility of this animal research being translated to humans. The original aim of the trial was to provide separate gestational environments for each developing shark that would otherwise be competing for resources as 'womb-mates', with an eye to using these tanks to prevent the cannibalistic stage of foetal development for the endangered grey nurse shark from further reducing the species numbers.[25] However, following media attention on the possibility the womb tanks could be adapted for human use, lead scientist, Nick Otway, responded that he had no plans to do this, stating: 'That might be possible, but I don't want to get into it because of the ethical issues … I'll stick with sharks.'[26] In 2024, Taketeru Tomita et al. published a paper in *MethodsX* detailing a 'portable-sized artificial uterine system for viviparous shark embryos', claiming their new model was only one-twentieth of the weight of previous designs, coming in at just 40 kilograms.[27] These two studies represent rare examples of non-mammalian animal experimentation in this space, with most other projects focused on using analogues for human infants. There is also increasing interest in using simulations to model how the relevant techniques for partial ectogenesis could be developed, aimed at achieving a user-centred design for the artificial womb itself.[28]

What is clear from the current state of the science of ectogenesis is that ethico-legal, rather than technical, issues may soon become the limiting factor in the development and release of this technology. As such, it is necessary to establish some of the ethical reasons justifying the promotion of this technology for use in humans, including its potential to promote health and sexual equality in reproduction. Exploring gendered issues of reproduction is also important when considering how the artificial womb might be fashioned and what uses might be supported in the future, as will be explored next.

Why sexual inequality in reproduction really matters

While the traditional African proverb 'it takes a village to raise a child' may well be right, it is still an inescapable fact of human biology that it takes an individual's body to grow one. According to Susan Rae Peterson: 'It is both a curse and a blessing that only women bear children. It is historically and economically a source of women's oppression. Yet the overwhelming significance of species survival through reproduction has guaranteed women a source of great potential power, power in the sense of ability rather than control.'[29] These conflicting views of power over reproduction lead to various contradictory feminist arguments regarding the potential for procreation to serve as a source of female empowerment or disempowerment. These carry with them various concerns regarding control over current and future assisted reproductive technologies, including ectogenesis. On the one hand, relieving women of the burdens of pregnancy and childbirth can be seen to promote greater sexual equality with men, who are not subject to the same burdens in human reproduction. This would challenge the foundation of many patriarchal systems that treat women differently based on their reproductive potential. On the other hand, removing women's unique influence over this aspect of human survival may lead to women becoming less valued in society, leading to further oppression. While the latter is a concern that demands careful consideration when introducing new reproductive technologies, the demands of the former justify the pursuit of alternative gestational options for women, such that they can reproduce without significantly greater risks or burdens than their male counterparts.

Referring to human reproduction as 'nature's traditional and bitter trap for the suppression of women', Mary O'Brien argues women's liberation depends on a thorough understanding of how this process works, biologically and socially.[30] Feminist philosopher Simone de Beauvoir similarly argues that women's social inferiority is due to the immanence of childbearing and the repressive social conditions women are relegated to under the guise of promoting family values and maternal instinct.[31] Challenging assumptions about women's 'natural' role in reproduction has the potential to liberate women from various forms of social and economic discrimination, with ectogenesis also opening up new possibilities for women who wish to have genetically related children without being pregnant or engaging a surrogate. This would yield benefits for both physiologically fertile and infertile women.

One of the major sources of inequality arising from sexual differences in reproduction is evidenced by the increasing social and legal restrictions on women's liberty while pregnant. Janice G. Raymond claims that doctors have now become 'police officers of pregnancy', reporting on behaviours of women that might harm their foetuses, rather than maintaining a primary focus on the health of their female patients.[32] She goes on to claim:

> Women are penalized for pregnancy. Equality in law is false, since the law does not recognize the real inequality that women face in law and in life for being pregnant, namely male dominance and female subordination, not to mention the physical toll and debilitation that many women experience during pregnancy.

> The point is not a biological one; it is profoundly social with legal implications. Only women get pregnant, and only women are subjected to discrimination on these grounds.[33]

While Raymond is correct in stating the major problem here is not a biological one, ectogenesis is still the only solution with the potential to both remove the 'physical toll' of pregnancy itself and challenge the very foundation of the social and legal discrimination against women due to their potential for pregnancy. Such discrimination manifests in many ways, but one example would be exclusion from certain occupations due to concerns about potential harm to foetuses from workplace exposures.[34] Ectogenesis would remove the threat of such exposure to foetuses, thereby also promoting the health and well-being of future children. Further examples of the restrictions women face as a result of their reproductive capacity will be addressed throughout the remainder of this chapter, including through the proliferation of so-called 'fetal abuse' laws.[35] With respect to sexual inequality in reproduction, it is particularly relevant that responsibility for foetal harm is so often attributed to individual women, despite what many consider to be the collective responsibility for risk factors, such as poor nutrition and housing, which often accompany extreme poverty.[36] When social disadvantage is the cause of poor foetal and infant well-being, yet individual women are still bearing the brunt of such recriminations, this provides evidence that sexual difference in reproduction easily translates to gender-based discrimination. Redressing the kinds of discrimination Raymond notes above certainly requires many social and legal interventions. However, even if we imagine a future in which such discrimination has been removed, women's reproductive autonomy would still be called into question by the lack of a genuine alternative to physical gestation.

Women's reproductive autonomy is also under threat through measures intended to limit access to contraceptives or abortion. Again, because women are the ones who get pregnant, such restrictions disproportionately impact women's health. In *Life's Dominion*, Ronald Dworkin argues that individuals have a right to 'control their own role in reproduction unless the state has a compelling reason for denying them that control', a position that is easy to defend when considering the uniquely personal nature of reproductive decisions and their connection to the culturally cherished goal of family creation.[37] However, when determining in what situations the state might have a sufficiently 'compelling' reason to interfere with reproductive liberty, women's disadvantage is compounded by the fact that they are typically under-represented in positions of political authority, including in most liberal democracies.[38] Christine Overall claims any legal and social system that effectively forces a woman to be pregnant against her will through lack of access to family planning measures makes women 'victims, through biological "destiny", of a sort of reproductive slavery'.[39] In terms of women's health outcomes, the psychological impact of diminished reproductive autonomy has been suggested as one of the major causes of the substantial differences in women's suicide rates across the globe.[40] For women's psychological well-being, it is essential that they are able to avoid or terminate unwanted pregnancies. In the absence of reliable contraception and access to safe abortion, a woman who does not wish to reproduce may be left with no choice but to be pregnant, a state that carries considerable psychological and physical risks. However, in the absence of ectogenesis, if a woman *does* wish to reproduce, she *also* may have no choice but to be pregnant, which often means subjecting herself to the various discriminatory practices outlined above. While the first scenario may be considered more serious, the core issue – an inability to avoid pregnancy while achieving one's desired family plans – is worthy of critical attention in both cases. Thus, the current goals of reproductive medicine appear to be based on a false dichotomy in which women are perceived to either wish to remain childless or to achieve a biological pregnancy. There is minimal attention paid to the reality that some women may wish to have biologically related children, but not gestate them. While some women will find surrogacy an acceptable alternative, many will not. Surrogacy arrangements also carry their own risks for prospective parents and, in many countries, are not legally enforceable for various ethico-legal reasons aimed at avoiding the potential exploitation and abuse of surrogates.

Compared with the restrictions placed on pregnant women, there is no equivalent loss of autonomy afflicting prospective fathers, minimal to no social or medical policing of their bodies and typically no physiological changes associated with reproduction impacting their health, freedom of movement or engagement in public life. But as O'Brien notes, borrowing from Jean-Jacques Rousseau, when it comes to reproductive labour 'men are "forced to be free"… [and] to be forced to be free is to render that freedom problematic'.[41] Sexual inequality in reproduction may be more obvious in the ways it disadvantages women, but it would be impolitic to assume that all prospective fathers are happy with the unequal division of reproductive labour. In the absence of technological alternatives to physical gestation, this forced freedom from pregnancy also means gay male couples are excluded from procreation without the assistance of a surrogate.[42] Thus, in addition to serving the interests of women who cannot or do not wish to be pregnant, ectogenesis has the potential to benefit prospective fathers. Rather than viewing this as a loss of power for women, it can be seen to represent a revolutionary attack on the maternal essentialism responsible for much of women's oppression related to reproduction. Importantly, pregnancy alternatives such as surrogacy and adoption still require that *a* woman is pregnant, even if she is not the intended mother. Unlike the male biological experience of reproduction, which carries no meaningful health risks, all current methods of gestating foetuses represent a significant burden for women.

The history of reproductive medicine and connections to science fiction

When it comes to predicting how the public will respond to ectogenesis, there are several lessons from the history of reproductive medicine that are worth considering. These also highlight why considering science-fictional representations of emerging technologies may be beneficial. This is particularly the case for technologies that might form part of the process of artificial gestation, such as IVF and humidicribs.[43] Despite some initial resistance, humidicribs have been widely embraced in neonatology as an effective means of saving the lives of infants born prematurely.[44] But here, the intersection of medicine and popular entertainment has yielded a disturbing example: the incubator-baby sideshows. These shows featured infants in humidicribs as medical curiosities in fairs across Europe and America between the 1890s and 1940s.[45] This concerning historical example is reflected in many visual representations of ectogenesis seen in various science fiction films, as will be addressed in the next chapter, where the visibility of the under-developed human foetus is treated as a gross spectacle.

Science fiction references also appear frequently in early discussions of IVF, with Gregory Pincus – the biologist who pioneered the first successful IVF pregnancy in rabbits in the 1930s – being labelled 'Dr Frankenstein' by *The New York Times*.[46] Similar slurs were also cast at Robert Edwards and Patrick Steptoe, the doctors involved in the first human IVF birth in 1978, which will be explored in more detail in Chapter 3.[47] Regarding ectogenesis specifically, there has always been a connection between this speculative technology and the field of science fiction. J. B. S. Haldane, often credited with coining the term in his lecture to the Heretics Society of the University of Cambridge in 1923, used a science-fictional narrative to explore the potential impacts of ectogenesis on future societies.[48] Following this, the idea of artificial human gestation gained notoriety through Aldous Huxley's popular dystopian classic, *Brave New World* (1932),[49] and various other science fiction narratives throughout the 1920s and 1930s.[50] Films like *The Island* (2004), *Man of Steel* (2013) and *The Matrix* franchise (1999–2021) all prominently feature ectogenesis, but the representation is mostly negative. A recent addition to this category, *The Pod Generation* (2023), has a somewhat more neutral representation of the technology itself but failed to impress audiences and critics or achieve the impact of these older examples. These and other cases are considered in more detail in Chapter 3.

Jay Clayton claims that 'the horrors of science fiction haunt the bioethical imagination', which goes some way towards explaining why the use of science-fictional references in bioethics tends to oppose technological development in the area of reproductive medicine.[51] Sarah DiGregorio also notes that due to its relationship with science fiction, real-world ectogenesis research has 'baggage', specifically citing associations with the 'battery farms in *The Matrix* or the hatcheries in *Brave New World*'.[52] Part of the reason this baggage exists is because both science fiction and emerging technology bioethics are inherently speculative genres of writing. As such, it is important to consider the role of imagination in bioethics to establish the significance of science fiction's relationship with this field of research. Before embarking on this journey, however, it is necessary to position ectogenesis in terms of both current scientific and bioethical scholarship.

The evolution of bioethics scholarship on ectogenesis

As demonstrated in the Introduction, historical arguments regarding ectogenesis tended to focus on women's liberation or oppression, either individually or collectively. However, following Partridge et al.'s announcement of the bio-bag trials in 2017, much of this scholarship has evolved to be more focused on foetal safety and the ethics of experimentation. This shift seems to imply a change of priority when considering a wholly hypothetical technology versus one that is now in prototyping. It also echoes cultural trends in various jurisdictions that are scaling back women's reproductive liberty in favour of granting rights to foetuses. While equity issues have always been featured in ectogenesis debates, the closer the technology comes to fruition, the more central these arguments have become as well. Concerns about the impact ectogenesis technology may have on abortion rights have remained consistent.

In 2023, the group responsible for the EXTEND bio-bag experiments published an article in *American Journal of Bioethics* (*AJOB*), entitled 'Ethics

Considerations Regarding Artificial Womb Technology for the Fetonate'.[53] This became a feature article inviting open peer commentaries, with the resulting responses providing a useful summary of much of the current bioethical thought on the subject. De Bie et al.'s article also contributed to the ongoing debate regarding what the entity growing in an artificial womb should be called, with these authors defending their choice of the portmanteau 'fetonate', meaning 'neonates kept in a fetal physiological state'.[54] This is intended to differentiate these neonatal intensive care unit (NICU) patients, who are receiving their nutrients and oxygenation via umbilical vessels in the artificial womb, from other premature infants receiving technological support in the form of conventional NICU incubation. The authors stress this distinction is a physiological one, rather than a moral or legal one.

According to De Bie et al., since their *Nature* article in 2017,[55] there have been more than thirty ethics articles published on the topic of artificial womb technology. However, these authors claim that 'most of these papers have focused on the very extreme and currently technically impossible use of AWT for "complete ectogenesis" (that is, the entire process from conception to birth occurring outside of a human body)'.[56] After considering several ethical concerns in the literature that they deem sufficiently 'reasonable' to warrant attention, the authors return to the topic of full ectogenesis, stating this concept represents 'nothing more than a technically and developmentally naïve, yet sensationally speculative, pipe dream'.[57] While it may certainly be politically expedient for scientists working on the artificial womb to distance themselves from what some consider the more controversial implications of their work, such dismissive pronouncements are difficult to accept at face value, as they match precisely those made regarding earlier reproductive technologies that have since become standard clinical practice. This point is raised in Seppe Segers and Dorian Accoe's response, where they state: 'Setting such scenarios aside as speculative "pipe dreams" may be an attempt to temper moral bewilderment and safeguard potential benefits. Yet, it is questionable whether merely expelling such views to the realm of science fiction will be sufficient to this end'.[58] These authors note that many of the concerns De Bie et al. raise as being overly speculative regarding ectogenesis are in fact already relevant in existing maternal healthcare, so relegating them to the realm of the fantastique is particularly problematic.[59] More importantly, however, De Bie et al.'s assertion that the distinction between full and partial ectogenesis is rarely made in bioethics scholarship is untrue, with many articles devoting significant time to comparing the two, as is seen in the various responses to De Bie et al.'s own paper, as well as many papers included in their scoping review. As will be explored in Chapter 3, the distinction is also sometimes present in science-fictional stories containing depictions of artificial gestation.

A summary of the current literature in ectogenesis ethics research includes the following elements: how candidates for artificial gestation should be selected (both during human trials and later in clinical practice); how these candidates can or should be extracted from the organic womb (in the case of partial ectogenesis); what terminology should be used for the candidates before, during and after extraction; what rights these candidates may have during the process; how these changes in terminology and rights may impact abortion rights; who should make decisions regarding these processes; and how can issues of inequity and inequality be managed in terms of access, affordability and potential discrimination. The remainder of this chapter addresses each of these issues in turn, using De Bie et al.'s article and its responses as a starting point. It then concludes by introducing how science fiction may help resolve some of the conceptual issues these debates expose. This strategy does not imply this specific *AJOB* collection contains all the relevant voices or recent arguments in this debate but rather recognizes the unique opportunity to review many key authors in the field responding to the *same* iteration of the technology in prototyping. As the collection was specifically curated to include the main concerns summarized above, as well as a diverse range of leading scholars focused on this technology, it provides an opportunity to explore a specific instance of emerging ectogenesis technology in the real world right at the moment where the scientists involved were seeking authorization to conduct 'first-in-human' trials. The following sections also situate the *AJOB* open peer commentary responses alongside other scholarship focused on each element to broaden the scope of the summary.

Current debates on the selection criteria for ectogenesis

On the issue of selecting candidates to trial the artificial womb, several authors suggest that early participation will be limited to those foetuses who would otherwise be expected to have very poor prognoses, particularly those at imminent risk of being born at twenty-two to twenty-four weeks' estimated gestation. For example, Tessa Gavina et al. suggested that experimental use of this technology would be 'exclusively tolerated by the medical community' in cases where alternatives carry a significant risk of morbidity and mortality for pregnant women and their offspring.[60] The same claims exist in older ectogenesis ethics literature, including as a solution to what Singer and Wells described as the 'catch 22' of trying to prove the safety of a new innovation by testing the unproven technology on vulnerable foetuses, something typically considered ethically unjustifiable.[61] The basic premise is that in cases where the foetus is almost certain to die or suffer significant disability otherwise, the moral threshold lowers such that the risks of foetal experimentation become tolerable.[62] However, Mark R. Mercurio and Kelly M. Werner note that 'gestational age alone is a poor proxy for prognosis' and claim that De Bie et al.'s cited data on survival rates for infants born at the above gestational ages were both outdated and biased.[63] Specifically, they note:

> The authors quote an overall survival at 22 weeks' gestation in 2012 of 9%, when more recent data show survival of 30–50% when resuscitation and intensive care are attempted. Survival at 23 weeks has, in recent years, been above 50%. … the potential benefit of AWT for any patient should be measured by the improved likelihood of a favorable outcome, *when compared to current aggressive treatment*. This promising technology need not, and should not, be oversold by reference to outdated or inapplicable outcomes data.[64]

If poor prognosis is to be one of the defining features justifying foetal experimentation, it seems reasonable to demand as accurate an estimation of this as possible. However, as Mercurio and Werner note, many statistics on survival following extremely premature birth include infants for whom 'no attempt was made' to preserve life.[65] E. J. Verweij and Elselijn Kingma also note the added complication that sometimes premature labour does not lead to imminent delivery, with the pregnancy instead continuing despite dire predictions to the contrary.[66] These authors are also particularly troubled by the potential for therapeutic misconception during early trials of partial ectogenesis, where trial participants 'mistakenly believe that research interventions are made on the basis of their individual therapeutic needs, rather than for research purposes'.[67] They claim:

> pregnant persons in disturbing situations are always looking for hope, and mothers will, and are socially strongly encouraged to, do anything necessary for their child to survive. It will be almost impossible not to escalate hope in this situation, and therefore doubtful that mothers who choose to participate … will do so in the (required) proper and full understanding that the aim of this research is the generation of future knowledge – not the rescuing of their child.[68]

Similar concerns about informed consent for ectogenesis research are discussed by John D. Lantos and Annie Janvier, who nevertheless accept that the only way to confirm that the results seen in animal studies can be replicated in humans is to conduct a formal clinical trial.[69] Montserrat Esquerda et al. suggest that determining appropriate inclusion criteria for such trials should be a priority, incorporating both technical requirements, such as health status and pregnancy type, and ethical requirements, including detailed risk/benefit analyses.[70] Writing for the *Journal of Perinatology*, Stephanie K. Kukora, George B. Mychaliska and Elliott Mark Weiss also stress an urgent need to establish clinically and ethically appropriate enrolment criteria for first-in-human trials for the various technologies classified as either an 'artificial placenta' or 'artificial womb', including establishing relevant scientific differences, comparisons of technologies and research ethics standards.[71] A related issue these authors note is inconsistency regarding these two terms and the systems they may describe.

There are also concerns in the literature regarding selecting candidates for artificial gestation after clinical trials have supported its integration into clinical practice. Again, Mercurio and Werner suggest just having a gestational age cut-off may not be appropriate, as foetal development is individual, and a 'relatively large' twenty-one-week foetus may stand to benefit from artificial gestation, even if the relevant hospital's policy is to deny access before, say, twenty two weeks.[72] These authors suggest 'strict lines of eligibility' may be easier to defend during clinical trials than in clinical practice in such a scenario, noting that 'should AWT become part of the clinical armamentarium', doctors will need to be 'prepared with an ethically defensible response' when refusing access to parents requesting it.[73] De Bie et al.'s framework suggests focusing on foetuses at twenty-two to twenty-five weeks' gestation, but Mercurio and Werner note that 'biology recognizes no such sharp lines of distinction'.[74] Similarly, Esquerda et al. claim that the gestational age limits proposed do not correspond to biological differences but technoscientific ones, which the artificial womb itself is set to modify.[75]

With the above discussions assuming ectogenesis availability only in cases of catastrophic pregnancy failure or extreme prematurity, criteria to access full ectogenesis are largely ignored. This is perhaps understandable, given the imminence of partial ectogenesis in society and the mere speculative possibility of anything beyond this. However, partial ectogenesis for non-emergency cases is considered in some responses to De Bie et al.'s framework, with James J. Cordeiro suggesting that elective use of the technology – for example, to resume usual work activities sooner – is morally impermissible due to the increased risk of foetal damage compared to continuing an otherwise healthy pregnancy.[76] Support for elective partial ectogenesis comes from a possibly unexpected source in the 2023 collection of writings though, with John Holmes and Laura Hosford suggesting Catholic doctrine could be interpreted in favour of this application of the technology.[77] Noting other Catholic writers, including Christopher Kaczor, have already defended the use of ectogenesis in obstetric emergency situations where the foetus' life is in danger,[78] these authors continue by appealing to the Catholic duty to 'participate in society and ... foster a healthy family' as grounds for women to use elective ectogenesis to meet their other social obligations, including promoting their career development as a means to better support their family.[79] No specific guidelines are suggested for what reasons might be given preference over others in the case that demand for elective partial ectogenesis outstrips supply. These authors do advocate for equitable access to the technology more broadly though, to promote other aspects of social justice and ensure its provision is ethically defensible within their faith tradition. Muhammad Ahmad Ibrahim AlJahsh similarly writes of a 'potential harmonisation between [AWT] and Islamic ethics',[80] drawing parallels to Marcia C. Inhorn's 2003 ethnographic studies focused on the acceptability of IVF practices for various Muslim traditions.[81] At the core of these religious arguments is a requirement that the technology be developed in a way that promotes the 'sanctity of life' and supports the family unit.

Current debates regarding foetal extraction

For those working on the science of ectogenesis, developing safe methods of transferring a foetus from an organic womb to an artificial womb represents a key challenge. As noted above, the ethical considerations of this process include who it should be offered to and why, but there are also other policy and ethico-legal concerns. De Bie et al. note that current assumptions include early delivery via caesarean (C-section), a procedure known to carry additional risks for the mother compared to vaginal delivery. However, these authors suggest many of these women would have been facing C-sections anyway, as candidates for artificial gestation are likely to be foetuses in distress, for which the likelihood of surgical delivery has already increased.[82] Nevertheless, they claim the decision to undergo foetal extraction via C-section to transfer a foetus to an artificial womb should be considered 'supererogatory', given the associated health risks for the mother.[83]

Tamara Kayali Browne et al. claim that the minimization of women's pain and suffering in discussions of foetal extraction via C-section speaks to broader issues of institutional sexism and obstetric violence.[84] Seppe Segers et al. have similarly noted that while increasing numbers of C-sections for supposedly non-medical reasons may 'create an image of Caesareans as minor interventions', there are some rare but very serious consequences, the risks of which should not be minimized.[85] Browne et al. also consider how full ectogenesis has the capacity to eliminate the embodied experience of pregnancy and birth, which for some pregnant people may mean losing a significant opportunity for bonding, while for others it may avoid traumatic birth experiences.[86] It is also noteworthy that it could produce both these results at the same time due to the highly individual and contextualized experience of reproduction for each person. That arguments against ectogenesis based on valorizing biological bonding risk alienating parents who are not biologically related to their children is also considered, particularly focused on the potential impact of this on adoptive and foster parents.[87] Seppe Segers and Elizabeth Chloe Romanis note that concerns with bonding may also apply in partial ectogenesis, given 'limited physical contact post-intervention', but they highlight that, to date, 'most attention in terms of (harmful) psychological effects, has been "offspring-centered", in which case it is hard to determine not only the scope of such presumed risks for the future child's psychological development, but also whether such concerns would be graver than the benefits that ectogestative technologies could bring'.[88] Overall, partial ectogenesis raises questions regarding how to safely and ethically extract a developing foetus from an organic womb, while full ectogenesis considers whether there are ethical issues with removing this stage of reproduction altogether. The latter point also speaks to concerns about defining 'birth' for entities that have been gestated artificially, as will be discussed later.

Verweij and Kingma have some concerns in common with Browne et al., including that 'it seems to be forgotten' that the patient at stake in early ectogenesis trials is the pregnant woman, stating: 'In first-in-human trials, she is the person whose consent should be sought. She will also be a direct patient–subject of the cesarean section currently deemed necessary to enable a transfer of the fetus.'[89] They call for risk proportionality when considering this process, such that it is only attempted when potential benefit to the foetus can reasonably be expected to 'outweigh the risks for the mother'.[90] However, the previously mentioned concerns regarding the mother's vulnerability and risk of therapeutic misconception still apply here.

Another substantive concern raised in response to the claim that foetal extraction methods will be 'controlled by the pregnant individual' comes from Susan Kennedy and Lawrence Nelson who note that in some jurisdictions foetal rights legislation has been used to deprive women of their civil liberties in reproductive matters, subjecting them to 'forced medical interventions, including C-sections, in an effort to promote the interests of the unborn'.[91] As such, these authors claim foetal extraction for subsequent artificial gestation may fall outside 'maternal autonomy' in legal practice, particularly in some parts of the United States.[92] Since the overturning of *Roe v Wade* (1973) by the US Supreme Court in 2022,[93] some states have enacted wide-ranging 'fetal personhood' laws that seem to substantiate this concern,[94] with Kennedy and Nelson claiming that women refusing to undergo foetal extraction in the future may face criminal charges for child neglect, endangerment or abuse, or be arrested and compelled to undergo the procedure if it is believed it may preserve the life or health of their foetus.[95] Far from being considered 'supererogatory', without proper protections, the advent of partial ectogenesis could be used by some to place additional moral and legal obligations on pregnant women to engage with this technology on the grounds of promoting foetal interests.[96] These concerns are echoed throughout the next two sections, which focus on the impact of ectogenesis on terminologies of pregnancies, foetal rights and abortion.

Current debates on ectogenesis terminology and foetal rights

For several years, bioethics articles on ectogenesis have often included a section justifying the authors' use of terminology. Elizabeth Chloe Romanis has advocated for the use of 'ectogestation' over 'ectogenesis' and 'gestateling' over 'fetus' or 'ectogenetic fetus', with the goal of capturing what is metaphysically unique about this form of gestation and the entity involved.[97] Lien De Proost and Geertjan Zuijdwegt related the use of 'perinate', 'ectogenic fetus' and 'prenatal human being' in the literature, while personally arguing that these novel terms have not 'helped to clarify the debate' about what the subject of the artificial womb fundamentally is, with De Bie et al.'s choice of 'fetonate' similarly dismissed.[98] These authors question the supposed need for new nomenclature, given '[i]n terms of physiology, scholars agree that the subject of AWT is a fetus', suggesting the entity should nevertheless be '*morally* treated as a neonate'.[99] They conclude:

> the subject of AWT is a fetus, but one that is treated as a neonate. To treat the subject of AWT as a neonate does not mean that it stops being a fetus, nor that it is a neonate. Ontological and moral status do not coincide, and common practices in public policy, medical care, and the lifeworld testify to the prevalence of this is-ought distinction.[100]

They further claim that the 'proliferation of terms' seen in recent ethics scholarship focused on ectogenesis is a result of issues surrounding abortion, rather than 'considerations germane to AWT'.[101] However, the use of the term 'artificial womb technology' has also been subject to criticism, with Verweij and Kingma claiming that bioethics scholarship has been misdirected by the 'widespread and misleading framing' of this technology as an artificial womb, instead proposing the 'more accurate (and less sensational) terminology "artificial amnion-and-placenta technology"'.[102] They reject any need to consider the implications of full ectogenesis on this terminology. One of the main reasons the more general terms 'ectogenesis' and 'artificial womb' are used in this book, however, is precisely to be inclusive of existing, future possible and even future impossible versions of this emerging technology, since many examples being analysed here only exist within speculative fiction and may never cross into the real world. As such, for the current project, the broadest terminological choices are most appropriate.

At its core, concerns about terminology are really a manifestation of concerns about moral and legal status. De Bie et al. downplay this issue by suggesting that a 'fetonate' would automatically be endowed with full legal rights and protections by nature of having been delivered alive from a uterus.[103] The reality is much more complicated though. Elselijn Kingma and Suki Finn have considered the significance of legal definitions of 'birth', suggesting the entity transferred from an organic womb while retaining its foetal physiology has been 'born-by-location-change' but not 'born-by-physiology-change', highlighting the difference between merely being delivered of the mother's body and being able to independently interact with the outside world.[104] Romanis summarizes this perspective as 'the subject of ex utero gestation has been *birthed*, meaning delivered from a pregnant person, but has not been *born*, meaning physiologically adapted to the external environment'.[105] She continues that, unlike a neonate, this entity lacks '"natality"/physical situatedness; it cannot be interacted with physically (held, touched, smelled) by the person(s) who intend to parent it.'[106] Romanis also considers the relationship between being *birthed, born* and the legally significant *born alive* when considering the novel situation of an entity that can have a 'temporary existence ex utero' before continuing foetal development.[107] Noting that the terminologies used to describe new biotechnologies can influence public reception of them, Esquerda et al. suggest a consensus on the definition of 'being born' may help clarify moral issues regarding ectogenesis in the same way that establishing criteria for brain death in 1969 settled various ethico-legal debates at that time.[108] Of the neologism 'fetonate', these authors question whether the term indicates a new entity or merely a new developmental situation for the existing foetus.[109] A proposal to define 'birth' as the permanent separation from a fluid-based gestational support system may help clarify the difference between continued gestation in an artificial womb and supported development through artificial incubation in the NICU; however, it is unlikely to appeal as a description of embodied pregnancy or the process of childbirth as a lived experience. This highlights the difficulty of developing consistent terms for processes that have biological and technological dimensions or manifestations.

What is ultimately at stake regarding terminological differences regarding gestation and birth is the matter of rights.[110] In many jurisdictions, a foetus has no rights, while a newborn possesses full human rights. Abortion is legal in many states, whereas infanticide is not. According to Leonard Michael Fleck, for those who argue that the *ex utero* foetus needs to be morally and practically treated as a neonate, discontinuing artificial gestation might therefore constitute 'gestaticide.'[111] Romanis considers these issues, suggesting an intuitive response may be to bestow more protection on an artificially gestating foetus than one *in utero*, because its life is not infringing on the liberty of another person, while also defending a position where ceasing the gestation of a 'gestateling' expected to suffer if it transitions to neonatal physiology may be morally permissible, even though actively ending the life of a suffering neonate may not.[112] Such inconsistencies are not radically different from ones that already exist in health law and policy, with De Proost and Zuijdwegt noting that in New Zealand, for example, liberal abortion laws co-exist with bereavement leave policies that can be accessed for spontaneous abortions (miscarriages), 'implying that the fetus is a person in law in one case, and not in another. … Inconsistency, it seems, is the hallmark of our dealings with fetuses.'[113] Kennedy and Nelson, however, are concerned about any conflation of moral and legal status for the entity involved in ectogenesis, accusing De Bie et al. of a 'less than accurate and incisive discussion of the law' as it pertains to potential future applications of their EXTEND platform, alongside a 'slipshod' discussion of the 'legal status of prematurely born infants and fetonates.'[114] Mercurio and Werner agree, stating: 'Despite the authors' statement that "fetonates" would be accorded the same rights and legal protections as other newborns, no laws currently protect the rights of fetonates.'[115] Again, De Proost and Zuijdwegt suggest the search for new terminology to describe this entity is less concerned with ontological differences and more with the moral status of foetuses more broadly, particularly with respect to the abortion debate, as will now be discussed.[116]

Current debates on abortion rights

Of the many potential ethical justifications for supporting abortion rights, one of the more common arguments rests on the right of a pregnant woman to refuse to have her body used to sustain the life of another being. Famously dramatized in Judith Jarvis Thomson's 1971 violinist thought experiment,[117] this argument posits that terminating a pregnancy is morally permissible as a means of exercising bodily autonomy and avoiding the physical, psychological, social and economic burdens of pregnancy, childbirth and childrearing. In most jurisdictions, there are gestational limits in place for accessing legal abortion, which may also differentiate between abortion on maternal request versus on medical grounds, for example, if the foetus is discovered to have a condition incompatible with life or the mother is experiencing a specific health threat. For laws that allow abortion on demand up until independent viability, reproductive biotechnologies have complicated and continue to complicate these limits. Ectogenesis continues this trend, with some arguing it may effectively remove the viability criteria altogether. As Eric Steiger notes, 'the fundamental point of ectogenesis is that it renders a fetus "viable", albeit with technological assistance, from the moment of fertilization'.[118] Here, he is discussing the potential for full ectogenesis; however, partial ectogenesis is still relevant when considering these ethico-legal boundaries. De Proost and Zuijdwegt suggest that the independence required to meet viability criteria should refer to 'independence from a human gestator', rather than independence from technological support, thereby limiting grounds for discontinuing artificial gestation once it has commenced.[119] Instead of these complications serving to oppose ectogenesis research, they can be taken as an opportunity to pre-empt these concerns and develop appropriate policies before the technology is released. As will be discussed in later chapters, this is one area where science-fictional visions of possible futures may be positioned to contribute to the integration of ectogenesis into society.

As demonstrated above, there are two distinct aspects of the abortion debate that are relevant to the current discussion: does the right to terminate a pregnancy include the right to terminate the life of the foetus, and under what grounds could an externalized pregnancy be terminated once appeals to bodily autonomy (arguably) no longer apply? For Thomson, the death of the foetus may be considered an unfortunate side effect of a woman exercising her right to an abortion – it is not the goal of the action, but the two events are inextricably linked.[120] Similarly, for those who only support abortion when there is a threat to the pregnant woman's life or health, a foetus in an artificial womb is unlikely to face this conflict. For the first question, providing the *option* of foetal extraction and subsequent artificial gestation when terminating a pregnancy seems relatively uncontroversial, assuming informed consent and technical suitability. Hendricks even suggests women experiencing unwanted pregnancies who have already decided to give the child up for adoption 'might prefer an earlier divestiture', using partial ectogenesis to achieve this goal.[121] What is usually of concern is the potential that once it is available, women will be *coerced* into this alternative when they would prefer to avoid genetic parenthood altogether. Joan C. Callahan and James W. Knight previously argued that abortion forms part of a pregnant woman's right to 'self-direction and bodily integrity', and that while she may choose to waive (voluntarily relinquish) this right, forced interventions for the sake of the foetus suggest pregnancy entails a forfeiture of this right, making pregnant women 'analogous to the criminal who can no longer demand that he or she not be interfered with by the state'.[122] Forced foetal extraction to avoid termination would similarly violate these rights. Those suggesting ectogenesis may one day serve as an alternative to all abortions also neglect the fact that the foetal extraction procedure is likely to remain far riskier than a standard termination of pregnancy and require the woman to stay pregnant for longer.[123] Since most abortions are conducted safely and easily in the early stages of pregnancy using medication, premature surgical delivery to transfer the foetus to an artificial womb instead is not an ethical substitute.[124] Nina Roesner also notes that since it is likely most pregnant women will be unable to access ectogenesis, leaving this as the only alternative to continuing an unwanted pregnancy will leave many with 'no options at all'.[125]

Opposing the perspective that ectogenesis might one day resolve the so-called 'pro-life' and 'pro-choice' political agendas, Joona Räsänen argues that the right to an abortion does entail the right to demand the death of the foetus, on the grounds of an individual's right 'not to become a biological parent, their rights to genetic privacy and their property rights'.[126] Since abortions are not just about not being pregnant anymore, providing an alternative to physical gestation does not satisfy all current uses or requirements. As such, ectogenesis does not provide an equivalent termination of pregnancy option and thus cannot replace the need for safe and legal abortion. Cannold's 1995 qualitative study found that women viewed abortion 'as a way to *prevent the creation* of something for which, once it comes into being, they will feel inescapably responsible'.[127] Seppe Segers claims abortion was seen in these cases as a method of 'motherhood prevention', while transferring the foetus into an artificial womb for subsequent adoption was not perceived to achieve the same objective.[128] In their response to De Bie et al.'s article, Benjamin Patterson Brown and Katie Watson similarly state:

> The perverse daydream of AWT as an abortion substitute also ignores the fact that the decision to create a new person in the world is a morally serious one, and people who have abortions are exercising their right to not reproduce.[129]

These authors suggest that while some seeking a termination of pregnancy may 'welcome an alternative that doesn't end in fetal demise', there should be 'vigilant separation' between such voluntary uses and any attempt to impose involuntary use, on the grounds that this would involve 'obvious subjugation of patient agency'.[130] More significantly, however, they argue that in jurisdictions currently able to 'force a pregnant person to be a walking womb against their will', ectogenesis is unlikely to be provided as an alternative since it represents 'an extremely expensive, less proven way to gestate'.[131] In other words, artificial gestation is not useful as a tool to placate the more vehemently anti-choice advocates in places where they already have the legal means of enforcing their agenda on others. This does not undermine the fact that it may have liberating potential for some who would choose it as an alternative to foeticidal pregnancy termination methods.

Accepting that there are elements of abortion that cannot be replaced by foetal extraction and transfer, the second question of what grounds may be used to justify terminating an *ex utero* gestation remains. Fleck rejects all Räsänen's arguments in this scenario, claiming that since the foetus in an artificial womb is in a 'public space' – for example, a NICU surrounded by health professionals – the 'right to privacy is irrelevant'.[132] Similarly, he states '[t]he property claim is also an ethical nonstarter' as foetuses and infants 'are not property in the way that cars and computers are property'.[133] The right not to become a biological parent may also be functionally irrelevant, depending on how 'birth' is ultimately defined. If the consensus ends up being that the entity inside an artificial womb should be considered a neonate, biological (and arguably social) parenthood already exists. Since such a foetus would not be imposing on another's body, Fleck claims that reasons for terminating artificial gestation 'would have to be ethically compelling'.[134] However, he also claims that 'all the nonvoluntary ethical justifications for an abortion would be entirely irrelevant: rape, incest, contraceptive failure, teen thoughtless sex, drunken sex, cannot afford another child, threat to the life or health of the mother, no right to use the mother's body'.[135] In reality, all of the above might be relevant as any one of these causes of impregnation may have occurred before transfer to the artificial womb.

For full ectogenesis, incest is still a possibility, and financial situations may change such that parents no longer feel able to provide for another child. As noted previously, the additional burden of having to undergo a C-section for foetal extraction means the bodily autonomy arguments stand as a reason for foregoing ectogenesis as an alternative to abortion. However, Fleck is correct that once the foetus is already out of the woman's body, such appeals are likely to be less compelling. This also introduces the perspective that when the foetus is no longer residing inside the mother's body, there is cause to distribute decision-making rights and responsibilities more equally across the parents. There is also the potential for future conflicts between biological and commissioning parents regarding who has decision-making responsibility for a foetus in an artificial womb destined for adoption, as will be considered in the next section.

Current debates on decision-making authority for ectogenesis

De Bie et al. suggest that once a foetus has been transferred into an artificial womb, 'decision making would become a shared parental responsibility and, for the majority of care decisions, both parents would need to agree'.[136] Family lawyers can presumably predict a wealth of cases arising from when couples separate during the gestation period and very much *do not agree* on the best way forward. Be that as it may, it is reasonable to expect a re-evaluation of parental decision-making authority once gestation is not tied so closely to the mother's body. Matteo Gulino et al. consider the suggestion that in cases where parents disagree about whether to access ectogenesis for their foetus, 'if the woman's body does not bring the fetus, there is no reason to regard the woman's wishes as overriding'.[137] Drawing analogies to other assisted reproductive services, such as IVF and surrogacy, these authors note there is a presumption that both commissioning parents provide consent, further suggesting that, since artificial gestation is currently experimental, the need for all parties to agree is even greater. Extrapolating from this point, they state: 'the two wills have the same value. … The NGP [non-gestating parent] has the decision-making power not because the fetonate has the same moral value as the newborn but because, if the fetus is outside the mother's body, the NGP and mother have the same value.'[138] However, these authors note this conclusion leads to ethically undesirable outcomes, diminishing the pregnant woman's autonomy by potentially forcing her to undergo foetal extraction procedures against her will, causing harm through obstetric violence and violating various justice principles.[139] This concern seems to bear out when considering Kyoko Takashima et al.'s commentary that suggests the choice to transfer a premature foetus to an artificial womb may sometimes constitute an 'ethical duty' or 'incomplete obligation' on behalf of the pregnant woman.[140] While they do not advocate for 'coercion or penalties by law' for failing to meet this ethical requirement, 'a relatively mild sanction such as moral blame by people around her' is supported.[141]

Another perspective on parental decision-making authority can be found in Steiger's 2010 article, 'Not of Woman Born: How Ectogenesis Will Change the Way We View Viability, Birth, and the Status of the Unborn', in which he argues:

> the unique strains and concerns placed on a woman during pregnancy create an interest in the naturally-developing fetus that supersedes both parents' property rights, and both the affirmative and negative procreative rights of the father. The interest is strong enough to justify complete control by the mother, including the right to unilaterally terminate, over a fetus developing naturally … If a fetus is growing ectogenetically, independent of its mother's body, then control over it must stem from her interest in it as a progenitor, which is equal to that of the father.[142]

Leaving aside that maternal and paternal genetic contributions are not in fact entirely equal, the above statement also assumes gestation will either be wholly organic or wholly artificial. The current progression of the science suggests that early use of ectogenesis will be limited to partial ectogenesis, necessitating a re-evaluation of the significance of *prior* gestation on decision-making authority over offspring. For full ectogenesis, the different methods for obtaining gametes may also challenge this presumption of equal authority; however, here the case is much stronger, thus demonstrating the equalizing potential of this technology.

Fleck concedes that a pregnant woman's bodily autonomy negates any right the genetic father may have to avoid parenthood by demanding an abortion. However, he suggests this restriction is eliminated once the foetus is externally located. Further, he claims that on separation, the foetus becomes the primary patient of NICU staff, thereby 'reduc[ing] considerably the decisional authority of parents'.[143] This is partly because the mother's own physical health is no longer intertwined and overriding. Gulino et al. claim that 'fetal viability and being outside the mother's body should be the two necessary conditions for giving the NGP the same decision-making power as the mother'.[144] Paradoxically, they also posit that since 'gestation is not part of male physiology', there are grounds to give women greater decision-making authority since, whether from conception or at some point during foetal development, the choice to use an artificial womb means the 'mother-to-be has renounced gestation'.[145] A scenario involving a conflict between two mothers-to-be using a sperm donor would be an interesting test case for this argument, as would any potential conflict between a surrogate and commissioning parents. Nevertheless, Gulino et al.'s suggestion does introduce an element few other commentators considered: that in replacing an *existing* process, artificial gestation may always be more linked to women's bodies even if no embodied pregnancy is ever involved. What has been *taken over* in this regard – gestation – has also been *taken from* a specific place/person. As will be considered in the final section of this chapter, the fact that a partially formed foetus was also formed from raw materials sourced inside the woman's body may also be a relevant factor.[146]

Current debates on equity and access to ectogenesis

Perhaps the most persistent ethical concern discussed throughout ectogenesis ethics scholarship is the issue of promoting equitable access to this technology. Continuing this discussion is essential to ensure that providing benefits for some women and prospective parents through ectogenesis services does not serve to diminish opportunities for others. Browne et al. relate that a common feminist concern regarding both full and partial ectogenesis is the possibility that it will lead to further marginalization of pregnant people by 'further shifting the responsibility of pregnancy and childbirth to a medicalized, technologically-controlled process'.[147] However, they also note the potential for greater equality in reproductive endeavours, including for women who 'have trouble conceiving or maintaining a pregnancy to term, and some LGBTIQ+ couples who cannot be co-biological parents', such as cis-gender gay male couples, and those who either cannot or do not wish to engage a surrogate.[148] Thus, these authors claim ectogenesis has 'queer reproductive potential', but this can only be realized if access policies are non-discriminatory, which has rarely been the case in assisted reproduction.[149] That full ectogenesis also has the potential to bring male and female contributions to human reproduction closer to equality is also considered.

Several respondents to De Bie et al.'s article accuse the authors of a lack of serious engagement with the social realities in which the artificial womb will function, including consideration of gender, race and class inequalities, and the impact of social attitudes toward different sexual orientations and family configurations.[150] In their commentary, 'Artificial Wombs or Artificial Feminism', Gavina et al.

suggest that the claim women may achieve greater 'competitiveness on the job market' if able to outsource (some part of) gestation 'unquestioningly accepts the framing of healthy bodies of women who are gestating as underperforming male bodies'.[151] Far from promoting gender equality in human reproduction, these authors suggest that such an argument 'shows a loyalty to the male standard that would compromise an author's ability to successfully advocate for women's rights'.[152] It also highlights another common equity concern, namely, that if ectogenesis is only available to wealthy women, *they* may experience greater employment competitiveness, but *other* women will suffer greater comparative disadvantage. A possible future in which employers can pressure women into foregoing biological gestation to avoid pregnancy-related illness and childbirth leave obligations is also invoked, as is a world where some women are deemed 'substandard gestators' that foetuses need to be protected from.[153] For the latter, Roesner claims this 'threatens to individualize and privatize broad social failures while ignoring the range of systemic factors responsible for poor and often disparate prenatal outcomes'.[154] As noted in previous sections, pregnant women are already facing greater sanctions for behaviours believed to harm their foetuses, and forced medical interventions are increasingly used as a method of promoting foetal interests over women's bodily autonomy.

Laura L. Kimberly and Gwendolyn P. Quinn are also concerned that the 'life-enhancing and potentially life-saving' potential of ectogenesis will be unfairly distributed on socio-economic grounds, noting there are already significant disparities in assisted reproductive technology access and outcomes in high- versus low-resource settings.[155] These authors note this is all the more concerning when considering that people from lower income communities tend to 'experience the highest rates of infertility along with lower quality health care'.[156] If ectogenesis were to be available only to wealthier citizens, this health disparity would likely increase as investment into maternity care would decline. Kimberly and Quinn also note similar disparities across heterosexual and LGBTIQ+ clients of assisted reproductive services, noting that '[p]eople who live in family configurations that do not conform to a traditional cisgender heteronormative nuclear family model often experience stigma and discrimination in family building attempts'.[157] Rather than opposing the release of novel ectogenesis technologies, these authors identify 'an opportunity to proactively integrate an inclusive, intersectional approach to fair access to AWT from the outset'.[158] It is precisely in this endeavour that this book hopes to identify a role for science fiction as a locus of the scientific imaginary and source of alternative visions of the future of reproduction.

What science fiction adds to the current debate

Of the eighteen open peer commentaries to the De Bie et al. article considered here, four directly reference science or speculative fiction, with two using the term as a pejorative to dismiss discussions of full ectogenesis at this time,[159] and the other two suggesting specific texts that may help readers contextualize De Bie et al.'s EXTEND experiments.[160] Of the former, what is perhaps most interesting is the comparison between these uses and Mercurio and Werner's claim that complete ectogenesis 'is a straw man – no technology enabling it is on the horizon, no one is seriously suggesting it anytime soon, and all ethical questions related to it certainly need not be settled before human trials of AWT begin'.[161] Within bioethics, and philosophy more broadly, the 'straw man' is an intentional exaggeration and misrepresentation of an opponent's argument to make it easier to dismiss, while the 'straw man fallacy' refers to the resultant refutation of an argument that is not actually the argument at stake. As will be demonstrated in later chapters, the use of science-fictional references in bioethics focused on ectogenesis often works to create a straw man by conflating the release of this technology with other supposedly undesirable outcomes. Nevertheless, the fact that 'science fiction' is a term used to denigrate certain arguments and their defenders within bioethics is worthy of note, especially given the existence of other well-established methods of achieving this goal in the field.

In discussing terminological differences, several commentators also highlight a potential use for speculative narratives when considering how words and labels can influence judgements about new technologies.[162] Science fiction authors have already trialled out various names for artificially gestated beings and explored how their treatment in society may differ according to the connotations attached to these terms, for example, the 'In Vitroes' from *Space: Above and Beyond* (1995–1996), who are sometimes derogatively called 'tanks' or 'nipple necks' in reference to the chambers they are gestated in and the umbilical port at the base of their necks.[163] These terms, and the visual differences these people display as a result of their artificial gestation, make them an easy target for discrimination. This visualization aspect is also relevant when considering other potential contributions of science fiction to the ectogenesis debate, as providing images and motifs of external foetal development could help bridge the gap in imagination regarding this emerging biotechnology. Roesner notes in her commentary that visualizing technologies have contributed to the over-medicalization of pregnancy and childbirth, 'leaving clinicians, rather than pregnant persons, as the experts on fetal wellbeing'.[164] Like various theorists to be discussed in the next chapter, Roesner links foetal imaging technologies to the 'conceptual separation of fetus and gestational mother [that] allows for maternal and fetal interests to be understood as adversarial', noting this has sometimes been used to 'justify overriding the decisions of fully capacitated pregnant persons to subject them to unwanted medical interventions'.[165] Thus, science fiction is positioned to explore both the battle of words (foetus, foetonate, gestateling, etc.) and the battle of images facing ectogenesis research, with consideration of how these may impact perception and social acceptance of this technology in the future. Science fiction can also construct alternative societies where speculative technologies have already been released, thereby dramatizing the common 'haves' and 'have nots' dilemma when it comes to distributive justice. By adopting points of view different to the reader's reality, it can also foster empathy for different perspectives. Each of these elements is considered in Chapter 2.

Science fiction also offers some specific representations of foetal extraction techniques that might help illustrate ethically salient points in this process. While it is unlikely anything akin to the 'fetal transporter' system used in *Star Trek: Voyager* to dematerialize a foetus from the womb and teleport it to an external incubator will ever be developed, a future where foetal transfer has become a 'routine out-patient procedure' is plausible, as is shown in David Weber's Honorverse series (the so-called tubing intervention).[166] How this might impact some of the above concerns about maternal bodily autonomy is currently unknown. There are also science-fictional narratives that directly compare the use of artificial wombs across cultures with liberal and restrictive abortion laws, such as Lois McMaster Bujold's *Shards of Honor* (1986), the first book of the Vorkosigan Saga.[167] This story also discusses how disagreements regarding terminating an artificial gestation might be handled in such a case.

Science fiction remains the only place where full ectogenesis is currently pictured, perhaps accounting for the lack of vision shown in some commentaries suggesting such an advance is impossible. What is clear from most of these statements is that the authors are extrapolating from the current partial ectogenesis trials and identifying that the components (e.g., pumps, tubes, etc.) could never be miniaturized to the point where they could serve a very early foetus. However, this ignores the potential for an artificial womb to be built from explanted uterine tissue or similar nutrient and blood-perfused material that allows organic placental development, modelling the process occurring in ectopic pregnancies. While these naturally occurring *ex utero* pregnancies are typically considered too dangerous to knowingly continue, in rare cases, viable offspring have been reported.[168] Even if it were impossible to sustain such a system for the entire length of gestation, it might help close some of the remaining gap between conception and the current partial ectogenesis prototypes.[169] Images of bioengineered wombs that are less dependent on synthetic tubes and tanks could also go some way toward demonstrating why bestowing equal parental authority over a partially formed foetus transferred to an artificial womb may not be as obvious a choice as several commentators have suggested. As Tim Bayne and Avery Kolers note, such a foetus would have been 'materially derived' from its gestational parent – literally constructed from nutrients obtained from the pregnant woman's body up until the point of extraction.[170] Using a closer analogue of biological gestation may more clearly demonstrate how, in embodied pregnancies, the foetus is making its demands of a specific person, rather than a machine. This could serve to further challenge the idea of the foetus and pregnant person as entirely separable entities. The more synthetic-looking artificial wombs fail to capitalize on this opportunity.

Regarding the two commentaries that specifically referenced science-fictional texts in their response to De Bie et al.'s target article, Leah Lomotey-Nakon and Elizabeth Lanphier note the radical potential of afrofuturist texts in particular to 'create worlds beyond contemporary configurations of injustices that consciously seek to disturb or dismantle the current configurations of the sociotechnical imaginary'.[171] These authors suggest studying works like Octavia E. Butler's Xenogenesis trilogy (1987–9) to explore the ethical dimensions of ectogenesis, stating:

> Afrofuturist and other visionary speculative fictions (VSF) are sociopolitical texts concerned with the futurity of nonwhite persons. … Through nonrealism, VSF uses defamiliarization and denaturalization as mechanisms of averting the reader's attention to the operations of oppressive powers.
>
> Other forms of bioethical discourse and methods of bioethical inquiry concerning technoscience, including case and policy analysis, critical histories of medicine as well as prophetic and anticipatory bioethics, diagnose and redress the operations of injustice using contemporary logics and ethical frameworks. Contrary to these approaches, visionary bioethics engages VSF as a method of discovering new moral landscapes and encouraging critical ethical reflection to reimagine the social worlds of medicine.[172]

This defamiliarization effect achieved by works of science fiction is discussed further in the next chapter under its related terms 'estrangement' and 'alienation', highlighting how ethical dilemmas can be abstracted from existing socio-cultural assumptions to explore what non-technological changes may be necessary to effectively integrate new technologies into society. For the above authors, this includes considering the racial implications of emerging reproductive biotechnologies. Similarly, Lantos and Janvier point to works like Helen Sedgwick's *The Growing Season* (2017) in their response, as a way of exploring concerns like those espoused by Corea regarding ectogenesis being used to replace women in patriarchal society.[173] Regarding human gestation more broadly, these authors state:

> Pregnancy is absolutely unique in ways that make analogies to other clinical or research situations inadequate. It is the only human situation in which two separate individuals are physically intertwined with one another. These biological facts demand a rich bioethical imagination.[174]

The next chapter explores this claim in detail, considering the role of imagination in bioethics and its possible contribution to the utopian impulse of promoting a world of sexual equality in human reproduction.

2

The role of imagination in bioethics

Many areas of bioethics are highly speculative, not only because they focus on future technologies but also because they consider how current practices in biology and medicine can and should be changed for ethical reasons. At their core, many bioethical arguments are exercises of the imagination, considering alternatives to the *status quo* for better or worse. Bioethics is also a highly interdisciplinary field, intersecting law, politics, science, medicine and philosophy. It is within the latter that the most work on imagination has been done, so this chapter will predominantly focus on philosophical theories of imagination. The purpose of this chapter is to explore the role of imagination in bioethics as a means of explaining how fictional representations of emerging technologies have come to play a role in this field of research. It will demonstrate that there is a special relationship between the field of bioethics and the science fiction genre in particular, which can be attributed to the fact that both are speculative, imaginative and narrative. They are speculative as they consider alternatives to our present and future, imaginative as they depend on an ability to creatively engage with these alternative realities to elucidate the possible consequences of each, and narrative as they both communicate and explore these consequences through the telling of stories and case studies. As such, it is appropriate to consider the intersection between these two fields through philosophical theories of the imagination and narratological analysis.

This chapter opens with a brief history of relevant philosophical theories about the imagination, proceeding to tie some of these theories to the concept of 'visual bioethics' and the better-known 'yuck factor' arguments in bioethics scholarship. The role of the moral emotions in bioethics and fiction will then be considered before an analysis of the narrative elements of the science fiction genre and the practice of bioethics. Together, these analyses open up a space where structure and form can be considered interpretatively, a theme which is then expanded in Chapter 3. Throughout these discussions, the likely impact of these elements of representation on public attitudes towards ectogenesis is considered.

Philosophical theories of imagination

In his book, *The Language of Imagination*, Alan R. White provides a useful overview of dominant philosophical theories of imagination. He begins with Aristotle and his successors – most notably René Descartes, George Berkeley, Thomas Hobbes and David Hume – claiming that for these philosophers to imagine something was to form a mental image of it.[1] He goes on to state for Descartes in particular, that which was 'not imageable' was considered 'unimaginable'.[2] In a letter to Mersenne in 1641, Descartes writes: 'whatever we conceive without an image is an idea of the pure mind, and whatever we conceive with an image is an idea of the imagination'.[3] Similarly, Berkeley limited the imaginable to the 'picturable'.[4] These philosophers relied heavily on the language of sight and visual experience to explain what the imagination was.

White claims that such image-based theories of imagination went out of favour in mainstream philosophy, partially due to their ableist dependence on the sense of sight. Tracing cultural theories of the senses from the Greeks through to modern Western culture, Martin Jay refers to such an impulse as 'ocularcentrism', noting the hierarchical placement of the 'distancing senses' of vision and hearing, above the more proximal senses of touch, taste and smell in many cultures.[5] However, forming visual and mental imagery still forms part of the common understanding of what it means to imagine the unfamiliar, opening up the possibility for film and art to make a substantial contribution to the imaginative work of bioethics, as such media provide visual images of things that may not exist in the real world and thus cannot be conceived in sense-perception through prior experience. Most notably for this chapter, this includes visualizations of artificial wombs and depictions of societies embracing ectogenesis as a means of reproduction. Such representations will be explored here with reference to a relatively underused method of bioethical analysis, Paul Lauritzen's 'visual bioethics'.[6] Focused on the ways images influence bioethical debate and perceptions of medicine more broadly, visual bioethics considers what bioethicists can learn from engaging with visual culture studies.[7] For the purposes of this argument, if imagining the future of human reproduction requires the formation of an associated mental image, emerging reproductive technologies rely on some mediating artefact to be imagined. For ectogenesis, this mediation may occur through adapting visual images of existing humidicribs or by engaging with mental images arising from fictional representations of the technology. The former is relatively straightforward, whereas the latter warrants closer attention, particularly given science fiction's fascination with ectogenesis.

Continuing his overview of philosophical theories of imagination, White claims that for Immanuel Kant, the imagination (*Einbildungskraft*) may do its work *through* imagery but can itself be distinguished from these mental images.[8] Fiona Hughes claims that for Kant, 'imagination transfigures the merely sensory given by directing to it a contemplative attention', such that it can stand in for intuition in the cognitive case.[9] The imagination is thus producing forms that can be apprehended and later assimilated into concepts for the understanding. These forms are often described as having image-like properties, but the imagination extends beyond these forms, creating a bridge to comprehension. Later philosophers, including Jean-Paul Sartre and Ludwig Wittgenstein, would abandon the 'imagist orthodoxy' altogether, arguing that mental images were not like pictures and that the association between the imagination and visual images had been misunderstood and was more about how imagination was *spoken of* than what it actually was.[10] For Wittgenstein, imagination was better conceived as a way of making sense of things when the facts of the real world failed to provide meaning.[11] In these, as in Kant's case, the imagination is being used to represent something otherwise intangible.

Both the image- and non-image-based theories of imagination are useful when considering methods of imagining the future of human reproduction. White notes: 'To imagine something is to *think of* it as possibly being so. It is usually also to think of it in a certain way'.[12] Thus, he claims imagination has a problem-solving purpose, as it allows us to consider hypothetical outcomes of our decisions and work through concerns regarding unfamiliar paths. When imagining what problems might need solving regarding the development and impact of new technologies, science-fictional worlds can provide a proxy for our own. In *The Seven Beauties of Science Fiction*, Istvan Csicsery-Ronay Jr. claims:

> It is from sf's thesaurus of images that we draw many of our metaphors and models for understanding our technologized world, and it is as sf that many of our impressions of technologically-aided desire and technology-riven anxiety are processed back into works of imagination.[13]

Science fiction is thus understood as a way to puzzle out what roles we want to allow new technologies to play in society and can even help disseminate information about scientific research currently being pursued.

It is in this latter capacity that Sheryl N. Hamilton claims science fiction has a crucial role to play 'as a mediator of biotechnological knowledge'.[14] As a locus of the scientific imaginary, works of science fiction not only depict new technologies and scientific achievements, they postulate how these changes will impact future societies.[15] If works of science fiction are helping construct models of the future, as Csicsery-Ronay suggests, bioethical analysis of science-fictional representations of reproduction and reproductive biotechnologies is needed. This is especially the case when considering technologies that currently only exist in the realm of futuristic fiction but need to be subjected to bioethical debate in the present, including ectogenesis.

Visual bioethics

In an article for the *American Journal of Bioethics* in 2008, Lauritzen implores bioethicists to consider the importance of 'visual bioethics', noting the rhetorical power, for example, of images of Dax Cowart's badly burned skin in discussions of patient autonomy, or the video ostensibly showing coma patient Terri Schiavo interacting with her parents as examples.[16] Through the first image, the abstract concept of non-consensual medical treatment can be concretized as a legitimate source of intense suffering, whereas in the second, fears regarding the possible uncertainty of diagnoses of brain death and subsequent cessation of life-sustaining treatment are brought to the fore. In both cases, these visualizations are powerfully persuasive. Lauritzen claims:

> despite the fact that images are ubiquitous and powerful, we have not, as a discipline, thought very carefully about how images function to persuade or move us, how arguments can take visual form – think of political cartoons – or how to deploy or evaluate images responsibly.[17]

With specific reference to the use of images to discuss reproductive ethics, Lauritzen draws on the 1984 anti-abortion film, *The Silent Scream*, as an example of 'emotional propaganda', which is verbally framed and 'visually mediated'.[18] His focus on the verbal narrative has led to some criticism from bioethicists, including Catherine Mills, for succumbing to the 'pull of language' rather than truly prioritizing the impact of the image alone.[19] Nevertheless, his analysis of *The Silent Scream* still yields some useful arguments, with Kathryn Woodward likewise considering this film a prime example of the importance of 'visualizing technologies' – in this case, ultrasonography – on representations of pregnant women and foetuses.[20] An important feminist concern since the 1980s, the ability to visualize a foetus *in utero* has significantly changed how pregnancy is, quite literally, viewed. Rosalind Petchesky claims that the abortion debates in the United States Congress during the 1980s were heavily influenced by the pro-life camp's usurpation of 'mass culture and imagery' to promote the foetus as a 'public presence'.[21] Noting the strategic use by anti-abortion groups of *The Silent Scream* film, and the public display of foetal remains alongside pronouncements that they 'sure *look like* a baby', Petchesky reflects on the lack of critical engagement with the authenticity, rather than relevance, of such images to the issue of a woman's right to choose.[22] Of particular interest is the complete erasure of pregnant women from these foetal images, even from their earliest appearance, an act Petchesky claims promotes the idea of the 'fetus as primary and autonomous, the woman as absent or peripheral'.[23] While such a representation is artificial and misleading, Suzanne Anker notes that even if a foetus *can* be considered to 'look like' a baby, this is not a morally relevant point. When discussing her foetal specimen art project with Sarah Franklin, she states: 'It looks like a baby. Is it a baby? No. It's not a baby. It's a never-been-born, un-dead specimen', a thing Franklin goes on to label a 'border entity'.[24] However, with the pregnant woman removed from view, this border entity can easily become the central focus.

For Woodward, the representation of the foetus as a victim in *The Silent Scream* is only possible through artful use of the foetal image:

> Women may be custodians of the image, but the mother's body is absent in the representation of the seemingly disembodied foetus, floating in space, suggesting an independent person, capable of separate existence. This counters the symbiotic relationship between mother and child, which was a feature of earlier, non-visual experiences based on feeling rather than seeing.[25]

These earlier representations of pregnancy she refers to were the subject of study for Barbara Duden, who discovered in the medical case records of an eighteenth-century German physician a dramatically different cultural understanding of pregnancy. She notes that in this era, a pregnancy was only confirmed after the mother reported feeling foetal movements (quickening), rather than through any medical testing. Before this event, there was no way to determine whether the symptoms of pregnancy being observed were the result of some other condition, such as a tumour.[26] Squier claims that now medical tests and ultrasound are used to confirm pregnancy, '[o]ne way of understanding the meaning of this shift from an emphasis on maternal testimony to a reliance on medical imaging and measurement is as a battle over representation'.[27] While the uterus was shielded from view in the absence of visualizing technologies, the mother and foetus could not be *imaged* separately and thus were not *imagined* separately. The pregnant woman's private experience of foetal movement could not be visually verified until parturition, when the resultant infant became a separate entity. The 'mass circulation' of foetal images facilitated through ultrasonography has constructed a common conception of the foetus as a 'free-floating' independent subject while still *in utero*.[28] This representation of the foetus permits consideration of foetal interests that may be in opposition to its mother, as is the case in films like *The Silent Scream*. Lynn M. Morgan and Meredith W. Michaels summarize this well in their introduction to 'Manipulating the Fetal Image' when they state:

> The ascendency of the fetus in recent years is directly tied to the circulation of fetal images. Though advances in visualization technologies have enabled the production of fetal images, their presence in our public and private lives is a result of their appropriation for specific social and political purposes.[29]

This quote recognizes that although reproductive technologies may be morally neutral in their own right, their use is often politically motivated. Likewise, the manicured foetal images that permeate the popular imagination serve a specific purpose within the right-to-life movement. Farquhar notes this 'imagery of the fetal astronaut', while linked to the medical technology that created it, 'relies on popular media for explication, dissemination, and endorsement'.[30] It is within this space that these otherwise neutral medical images are overlaid with cultural meaning, including bestowing 'fetal personhood' through visualization.[31]

Sonogram images may be used in the real world to promote an idealized image of the foetus as a supposedly independent subject. Such a representation of the foetal entity promotes the idea that a developing foetus is worthy of moral consideration, even when this may cause a conflict with respecting the rights of the pregnant woman within whom the foetus resides. However, when similar images of a stand-alone foetus are used in the context of ectogenesis, the intended result is often to invoke feelings of horror or disgust, rather than concern for the foetus. The free-floating foetal image that so helpfully erased the physical existence of the gestating woman in the first instance is now, in the genuine absence of a woman's body, a source of discomfort. This chapter will now explore this potential contradiction, using two leading examples from science fiction film – *The Island* (2005) and *The Matrix* (1999) – and applying Lauritzen's theory of visual bioethics. Where these two films sit within science fiction's treatment of ectogenesis more broadly will be discussed in the next chapter.

Applying visual bioethics to ectogenesis in science fiction

Assisting in the visualization of unrealized futures and technologies is one of the primary contributions science fiction can make to bioethical debate; however, as will be explored throughout the remainder of this book, the pattern of representation in the case of ectogenesis is far from neutral. Take the example of *The Island* (2005), in which human clones are grown in ectogenesis pods to provide autologous 'spare parts' for wealthy clients. These clones are matured in massive tanks until 'birth', with the film including various images focused on the dehumanizing experience of being brought into the world this way. The clones are then housed in a compound where they are systematically lied to in order to keep them from trying to escape into the outside world. Told that Earth suffered a catastrophic disaster and that there is only one habitable region left – the Island – the clones await the daily 'lottery' to see if they have been chosen to go there. In reality, the names selected represent the clones about to have their organs harvested. These human clones have been denied a unique identity, not only because they are genetically identical to the clients who commissioned them but also because they were mass-produced. The birth scene in the film is particularly distasteful, with one of the characters complaining that he will be sick if he has to witness the event. As the ectogenesis pod is sliced open, amniotic fluid gushes out, and the camera focuses on one of the technician's shoes being drenched in the viscous substance. Immediately before this scene, the artificial umbilical cord was severed, causing blood to spurt out from the site and ooze slowly down the side of the pod. Again, the camera zooms in on this fluid, and the audience gets a sense of the unpleasant stickiness that later requires the whole delivery suite to be hosed clean. At the end of the birth scene, a physician arrives to assess the clone's health, declaring: 'It looks like we have a fine product'.[32] It is unclear whether the same revulsion would be felt about a natural (e.g., non-clone) delivery – as there are none depicted in the film – but there is no ambiguity regarding how distasteful this birth scene is.

This visual representation captures how alien the clones' gestation and delivery are, how far removed from the biological norm. This is primarily achieved through the exaggeration of natural processes, including waters breaking and postpartum bleeding, which are filmed in such a way as to ensure the audience is disgusted by the scene before them. In his book *Daedalus: Science and the Future*, Haldane notes that technologies like ectogenesis are often considered 'perversions' of biology, appearing 'indecent and unnatural'.[33] This is certainly the case in *The Island*, where the birth scene is a grotesque imitation of natural childbirth. Nick Bostrom considers Haldane's discussion of concerns regarding ectogenesis as an early articulation of the 'yuck factor' objection to reproductive biotechnology.[34] This argument suggests that when people are repulsed by something, irrespective of whether their reaction is logical, this suggests there is something morally repugnant about the object of their disgust. Sara Ahmed notes that disgust is not an abstract experience, but an 'intense bodily feeling of being sickened' that is always directed towards a specific, repellent object.[35] As full ectogenesis chambers are not objects that actually exist, any attachment of feelings of disgust must be to the idea or image of this future technology. In this, the birth scene from *The Island* provides a useful substitute for the real thing. While nature dictates that loss of bodily fluids accompanies the expulsion of progeny from the womb, there is no such imperative present in a controlled laboratory environment. Even less so when considering this delivery suite is entirely fictional. Thus, the choice to have fluids gushing to the floor in this scene is just that: *a choice*, and one that can successfully invoke feelings of disgust in the audience.

However, it is not just that these clones are artificially grown and delivered that renders their births potentially revolting. Another 'exaggeration' of the natural birth process is that they are born as adults. Unlike in most cases, infants are only indirectly created using ectogenesis technology in this film. As such, one particularly interesting element of the treatment of ectogenesis in *The Island* relates to surrogacy. Instead of growing babies ectogenetically for wealthy clients, or simply allowing them to engage gestational surrogates in the usual manner, clones of the women are grown and used as surrogates to gestate their genetic offspring. Within the compound, going into labour is celebrated, as this is known to automatically lead to a transfer to the Island. The horror of being killed for body parts is then mirrored in the 'termination' of surrogacy contracts, such as when the character, Lima One Alpha, receives a lethal injection shortly after giving birth. As a business model, it must be noted that this policy is highly ineffective; first, because it presumably wastes the surrogate's valuable organs; and second, because other female clones could just as well serve as gestational surrogates, leaving no need to grow these particular clones. However, the possibility of gestating humans beyond the infant stage – for example, to produce clone surrogates – is the only element of the film that truly necessitates extra-corporeal gestation. It seems that while the film is willing to depict an unnatural 'product' of an unnatural 'birth' – evidenced by both the adult states of the clones and the lack of any female characters involved in their delivery – it is unwilling to show ectogenetically grown babies. Whether such a vision was deemed *too* revolting to include can only be speculated on, but it is noteworthy that one of the more significant plot holes in the movie has come about through its active avoidance.

The representation of ectogenesis in *The Matrix* (1999) further exaggerates the potentially 'disgusting' elements of this method of procreating. In this film, robots have taken over the planet and are using humans as a source of electrical energy. Artificial gestation keeps the human population growing, with visually disturbing scenes showing rows of incubation pods covered with grime and spider-like machines crawling over the developing foetuses. There is no other reason for these artificial arachnids to exist in the film except to repulse the audience. By contrast, those born through an organic womb outside of the simulated world humans have been enslaved in are considered superior, with the character Tank explaining his lack of ectogenesis plug 'holes', saying: 'Holes? Nope. Me and my brother Dozer, we're both one hundred percent pure, old fashioned, home-grown human, born free right here in the real world. Genuine child of Zion'.[36] However, while Tank may be more 'genuine', he is not the star of the show. In the case of *The Matrix*, the protagonist, Neo, is the character audiences are most positioned to support. As with the example from *The Island*, when Neo is extracted from his artificial womb, the visual imagery focuses on the displacement of fluid and violent disconnection of life support systems. Whatever else the audience gleans from this scene, Neo's near-drowning in synthetic amniotic fluid is threatening and revolting.

Visual bioethics meets the 'Yuck Factor'

As noted above, the visualizations of artificial gestation provided in science fiction often aim at achieving a feeling of revulsion in audiences. This is where visual bioethics intersects with an older tradition in bioethics scholarship: articulations of the 'yuck factor'. In his famous article 'The Wisdom of Repugnance', Leon Kass argues, 'repugnance is the emotional expression of deep wisdom, beyond reason's power to fully articulate it'.[37] However, even he admits that 'revulsion is not an argument' and that what disgusted society in the past may not be considered disgusting now.[38] As can be seen in the descriptions above, any moral repugnance the audience may already feel towards artificial wombs can be exacerbated by the depictions of the technology in these films. Lauritzen notes that film is a particularly persuasive medium, as not only are there visual cues to excite the imagination, but there is 'an interplay of words and images' provided through the narration.[39] Of particular interest when considering both *The Island* and *The Matrix* is the fact that while the ectogenesis scenes are given a lot of visual attention, artificial gestation is not required for the plot of either text. In fact, a study of the use of ectogenesis in science fiction yields very few examples in which the narrative depends on the technology for coherence. As such, the choice to depict ectogenesis in this way does not advance the overarching plot of either story; however, it may succeed in eliciting a visceral reaction in the audience. One obvious reason for the above visual treatment is that many of the surrounding socio-political 'horrors' of these texts cannot be easily pictured. Thus, the negative imagery of ectogenesis is providing a locus for the audience's disgust against the various undesirable aspects of the fictional worlds shown, such as exploitation of the disadvantaged. However, this practice risks conflating the issues associated with ectogenesis with those often more substantive problems, such as slavery, extreme inequality and human reproductive cloning.

Julia Kristeva's theory of abjection has clear relevance to the 'yuck factor' as it functions in bioethics. According to this theory, the feelings of revulsion one may have when faced with the abject are not due to anything genuinely unclean or defiling, but rather are a reaction to a perceived threat to identity, established systems and order.[40] For Kristeva, the unfamiliar abject 'does not respect borders, positions, rules', while its opposite ritualizes social prohibitions, valorizes the symbolic purity of the mother figure in society and justifies the separation of the sexes, placing men in power over women.[41] That visions of ectogenesis often find themselves on the wrong side of this equation is not altogether surprising, since they represent a disruption to many of the above social norms. Philip Ball claims that while some people will be accepting of ectogenesis in the real world, '[o]thers will never be convinced that there is a place for an artificial womb. To the extent that this is a visceral response, it should not be rejected out of hand as a triumph of sentiment over reason: visceral responses may have their reasons too.'[42] By this logic, just because the 'yuck factor' is easily exploited does not mean that it should be disregarded entirely. Nevertheless, awareness of the potential to exacerbate existing fears through such tactics should be met with restraint, ensuring that the threshold for persuasive argument is not diminished by appealing to feelings of revulsion toward the unfamiliar. With regard to the influence of science fiction in bioethics, a vicious cycle can arise in which science fiction authors find inspiration in contemporary concerns about emerging technologies, but their works later serve to fuel conservative objections to these developments in the future. Evidence of this impact can be found in the frequency with which bioethics scholarship references texts like *Frankenstein*

(1818) and *Brave New World* (1932), both of which serve as cautionary tales regarding the integration of scientific advancement into society.

The role of emotion in moral spectatorship

Moving beyond feelings of disgust and the purely visual aspects of imagination opens up a wider discussion of the use of affect in bioethical debate. This provides a space for both visual and non-image-based art forms, such as literature, to contribute to the act of imagining. Northrop Frye claims that narrative storytelling is a form of 'imaginative basic training', an active process by which we learn to consider alternative experiences.[43] The visceral response to science fiction imagery of possible reproductive futures is only one method by which consumers of these narratives may be influenced by science fiction's engagement with bioethical issues. Another major opportunity arises from emotional involvement with the fictional characters depicted in science fiction.

In her book *Moral Spectatorship*, Lisa Cartwright claims: 'Little has been said about how screen characters are constituted as viable and compelling models of human subjecthood with which spectators might identify'.[44] The same can be said for fictional characters in literature. The identification between the reader and the character is essential for fiction to achieve its potential for ethical instruction. Evelyn Tsitas claims writers of fiction make bioethical issues 'flesh and blood through imaginary characters and their plight', making the reader or viewer 'feel and care' about the human aspect of the issue.[45] The power of fictional narratives in engaging the public on bioethical issues rests in part with the writer's ability to make the audience identify and empathize with the characters in the story, highlighting that bioethical dilemmas always impact human relationships. In contrast to the depersonalized clinical vignettes that typically occupy the bioethics classroom, fictional characters from film and literature are often *designed* to encourage emotional attachment. This challenges the primacy of universalism and rationality when contemplating bioethical issues by considering the contribution of emotional engagement.

For Sheila Jasanoff, what is lacking in science and technology studies scholarship when considering the impact of emerging technologies are the 'conceptual frameworks that situate technologies within the integrated material, moral, and social landscapes that science fiction offers up in such abundance'.[46] This same lack of diversity can often be found in bioethics literature considering ectogenesis, either through introducing this new technology with rigid adherence to maintaining current socio-political institutions or through insistence that the introduction of this new technology would inevitably lead to a total collapse of these same systems. Thus, the ability to explore the potential social implications of technologies on human relationships is a major strength of science fiction in bioethical debate, as it provides the opportunity to consider future worlds in which ectogenesis has been successfully or unsuccessfully integrated into an altered society and what other changes contributed to this result. Jasanoff also notes that technological achievements typically lag behind 'authorial imagination by decades or longer', indicating an opportunity to consider these issues in advance of the technology being developed and released.[47] Such considerations may include the logistical and emotional ramifications of technological change.

According to Colin Radford and Michael Weston, philosophers have long been troubled by the inconsistency of humans feeling genuine emotion for fictional characters while simultaneously lacking empathy for the real suffering of others. Using the death of Mercutio in Shakespeare's *Romeo and Juliet* as an example, these authors note:

> we cannot say that we do not feel for fictional characters, that we are not sometimes moved by what happens to them. We shed real tears for Mercutio. They are not crocodile tears, they are dragged from us and they are not the sort of tears that are produced by cigarette smoke in the theatre. There is a lump in our throats, and it's not the sort of lump that is produced by swallowing a fishbone.[48]

Despite providing eight alternative arguments to account for this emotional reaction, the authors conclude that while the phenomenon is inescapably real, it may not be rationally explainable. If the audience is sufficiently 'caught up' in the story, they are capable of feeling real emotion for characters that they never forget are fictional.[49] As such, promoting emotional engagement with certain characters in a narrative might plausibly have a flow-on effect when it comes to moral judgements about the fictional world those characters inhabit. If positioned to pity the clones in *The Island*, audiences are likewise positioned to chastise the fictional doctors who created them. If repulsed by Neo's 'birth' but unable to blame him for this feeling, the disgust must be attached to the object involved in the scene, rather than the person. These interpretive choices are both cognitive and emotional.

While it may not be the intention of a science fiction author to persuade an audience of a particular moral argument, Daniel Jacobson outlines various ways in which engaging the reader's emotions through narrative can have an ethical impact. Beginning with Horace's famous claim that poets should 'please or instruct', Jacobson goes on to show that aesthetic cognitivism (the belief that the most valuable aspect of art is the knowledge gained from it) is not limited by authorial intention to provide moral instruction. Rather, he claims from the outset: 'it is crucial to recognize that art can serve an ethical function without its manifesting didactic intentions and moralistic purposes'.[50] He later continues this argument by stating:

> My proposal is that the primary ethical function of narrative art is to provide imaginative acquaintance with the ethical perspectives which works of narrative art characteristically trade in, but may or may not advocate. This *acquaintance* model is compatible with poetic assertion, but it does not require it; we can learn from a work without being taught by it. Hence it is not biased toward didactic works or propaganda.[51]

He claims exposure to different ethical perspectives involves emotional engagement and enhanced 'perceptual capacity', such that when sympathizing with a fictional character, one can be convinced this is an appropriate feeling to experience.[52] In science fiction narratives involving future reproductive technologies, the characters the audience are positioned to sympathize with is significant when it comes to moral instruction regarding the technology.

As a final consideration, Noël Carroll claims that common objections to the proposed value of literature in philosophical debates include that such stories are banal, lack evidence or lack argument.[53] He continues by establishing an analogy between narrative fictions and the narrative and fictional thought experiments typically used in philosophy that are not rejected on these grounds, noting that fiction functions in the same way but for a wider audience than just moral philosophers.[54] As this book proposes using various analytical techniques, including narratological methodology, to enhance the constructive relationship between bioethics and science fiction, the remainder of this chapter will focus on how both of these fields can be defined as narrative genres suited to such analysis.

Science fiction as a narrative genre

Defining the science fiction genre is notoriously difficult. This is in large part due to the slippery nature of such genre definitions, particularly when applied to a form typically thought to encompass film, literature and graphic novels, and which might also be attached to certain works of art, music and expressions of fan culture. While it is not the intention of this section to create yet another prescription for the genre, to apply narratological and other methods of literary analysis to 'science fiction', it is first necessary to establish some proposed boundaries for what might reasonably be included within this narrative genre.

One of the more defeatist methods of dealing with the issue of delimiting the field of science fiction is to avoid trying to define it at all. For Paul Kincaid, there can be no firm definition or starting point for the genre, 'no ancestral text that could possibly contain, even in nascent form, all that we have come to identify as science fiction'.[55] He notes that Gary K. Wolfe's seminal work on science fiction scholarship alone lists thirty-three overlapping and contradictory definitions, claiming that various scholars seem almost obsessed with capturing the 'first' example of the genre. Some date the beginnings of the genre with Thomas More's *Utopia* (1516), others consider Mary Shelley's horror classic *Frankenstein; or, the Modern Prometheus* (1818) to be the first science fiction text.[56] For Kincaid, such efforts at establishing the true origin of the genre are fruitless as '[w]hat part of Frankenstein, for instance, as diluted as homeopathic medicine, is to be found in Philip K. Dick's *The Martian Timeslip*, or Gene Wolfe's *The Book of the New Sun*?'[57] Similarly, for Matthew Cheney, a definition of science fiction is impossible '[b]ecause SF relies on *difference*, it cannot be stuck in a static structure such as a comprehensive definition'.[58] Some critics even suggest that rather than being a genre in its own right, science fiction is better described as a 'substantive topic' predominantly concerned with speculation.[59] For obvious reasons, this method is not very practically useful, so alternatives must be sought.

For other science fiction scholars, such as Samuel R. Delany, genre classification is more about reader responses and marketing than any inherent properties of the text. Providing as an example the phrase 'He turned on his left side', Delany claims that an audience primed to receive this phrase in a naturalist sense might imagine a man turning in his bed, whereas an audience encountering this same phrase in a science-fictional text may conceive of someone literally switching on the power to the left side of their body.[60] Thus, Delany claims 'we read words differently when we read them as science fiction'.[61] What is important here is considering what avenues for the imagination are opened up in science fiction, which may not be available for audiences of other genres, such as realist or fantasy fiction. In his article, 'On Defining SF, or Not: Genre Theory, SF, and History', John Rieder notes of Delany's example:

> the second reading depends upon the reader's familiarity with and use of sf conventions – in particular, here, the expectation that the distinction between organism and machine is going to be blurred or violated. Both the writer and the

> reader of the sentence in its sf sense are using the genre to actively shape their understanding of the world.[62]

However, shifting the focus onto audience identification leaves some scholars with no more prescriptive boundary for science fiction than that readers report a particular text 'feels like science fiction'.[63] Borrowing from Wittgenstein, such scholars argue there is a 'family resemblance' between texts of the science fiction genre, which allows the audience to group the works together based on a range of characteristics, rather than a 'single shared defining element'.[64] These characteristics might include interstellar travel, a technological development, a utopian society or a future setting, to name a few.[65] For the current project, the mere inclusion of a speculative reproductive technology, such as full ectogenesis, might satisfy the requirement. When considering that many science fiction texts bear very little resemblance to each other, Rieder claims that the notion of the 'fuzzy set' from mathematics also provides a useful conceptual model for the genre, in which membership into the set can be based on various levels of intensity, with some elements containing many relevant characteristics, while others may contain only one.[66] As such, any two texts within the genre may share no relevant properties in common, while still both being identifiable as science fiction. This is important from a marketing perspective, as genres represent a sort of contract between authors, publishers and consumers, influencing who will purchase a text and how they are primed to respond to it. Though again, this method does not provide reliable inclusion or exclusion criteria for potential science fiction texts.

When considering Raymond Williams' notion of 'selective traditions', Andrew Milner notes that both the search for an ancestral text and the concept of a 'family resemblance' may fail in their goal of defining science fiction as a genre:

> Genre is also tradition, and traditions are, as Raymond Williams notes, necessarily selective – that is, they are forged through a continuously changing competitive struggle to select and re-select one's own cultural ancestors. The passivity of the notion of the family resemblance renders it incapable of explaining what is most characteristic of selective traditions, that is, their selectivity.[67]

Milner sees the 'plethora of well-known "Definitions of SF"' available online and in science fiction criticism as evidence of this continuous struggle. He does, however, point to one 'selection' that provides the kind of prescriptive genre boundary desired for this analysis, the one put forward by science fiction scholar, Darko Suvin, in 1978.[68]

Generally considered to be the most influential definition of the genre, and the one that provides the most useful guidance for this project, Suvin defined science fiction as the 'literature of estrangement', also claiming that '*SF is distinguished by the narrative dominance of a fictional novelty* (*novum*, innovation) *validated by … cognitive logic*'.[69] By this, he meant that although the worlds of science fiction are different from our empirical universe, what happens there must make some logical sense relative to the accepted knowledge of the time.[70] For Suvin, any acknowledgement of 'metaphysical agency' – for example, the use of magic or religious mythology – automatically disqualifies a text from the science fiction genre, because such elements cannot be validated through 'scientifically methodical cognition'.[71] Thus, the 'estrangement' occurs as the reader is transported to an unfamiliar environment where they experience feelings of alienation and not through the exploration of alternative realities that go 'beyond the ideal possibilities of physics or any other science'.[72] Suvin's use of this term 'estrangement' relates to Bertolt Brecht's *Verfremdungseffekt*, or V-effekt (variably translated as the 'estrangement-effect', or 'alienation-effect'). As in Brechtian theatre, Suvin's concept of estrangement refers to the audience being denied the comfort of a timeless and 'naturalist' reading, instead being constantly reminded that what they are experiencing is historicized, changeable and, most importantly, distanced from reality. In short, neither the reader of science fiction nor the viewer of Brechtian theatre is permitted to forget that they are witnessing a fiction. As noted by Fredric Jameson, and relevant to Suvin's Marxist agenda for science fiction, reminding the reader that what they are reading has been 'constructed by humans' simultaneously communicates that it can be re-constructed or replaced by humans as well.[73] This is particularly relevant for utopian literature, as will be discussed later.

Suvin's definition of 'significant' science fiction further specifies that works should focus on the 'political, psychological, and anthropological *use and effect of knowledge*' to fulfil its function as a subversive genre.[74] Gregory Renault explains Suvin's argument by stating: 'The claim is that naturalist fiction portrays the Same (author's empirical environment) by the Same ("exact recreation"), while estranged fiction, such as science fiction, portrays the Same by the Other', and in so doing provides 'both a reflection and a critique of society'.[75] While Suvin was primarily interested in science fiction literature, his definition also works well for science fiction film. For texts involving alternative methods of reproduction and family-making, the critique is often focused on what is happening in society today that could promote or frustrate the realization of this alternative socio-technical system.

There have been various attempts to refine Suvin's definition of science fiction, including a proposal by Carl Freedman to replace 'cognitive estrangement' with the 'cognition effect'. Noting the difficulties of engaging literary analysis for a genre in which there remains no 'definitional consensus' among scholars, Freedman continues by claiming that Suvin's definition remains 'not only fundamentally sound but indispensable'.[76] However, he argues that Suvin's dependence on 'scientifically methodical cognition' effectively renders the science fiction label dependent on 'epistemological judgment external to the text itself' and, in particular, judgements regarding the continued plausibility of the technoscience imagined.[77] Using Isaac Asimov's 'The Dying Night' (1956) as an example, Freedman claims that the need for validation by 'cognitive logic' would retrospectively disqualify this text from the science fiction genre, since its narrative coherence depends on a plot device – namely, the captured rotation of the planet, Mercury – whose scientific validity was later debunked.[78] Freedman claims this issue can be avoided by relying instead on the text's ability to achieve a 'cognition effect', best described by China Miéville as a reliance 'not on the language of science, nor on the command of that language, but on the *appearance* of that command … *something done with language by someone to someone*'.[79] For Miéville, the cognition effect persuades the reader, through '*charismatic authority*', to accept the estranging, science-like qualities of the text, without relying on actual scientific validity.[80] In this way, incorrectly described science, such as Asimov's description of Mercury's rotation, or even the inclusion of various pseudosciences, need not pose an obstacle to classification as science fiction. Mark Bould notes the usefulness of this new criterion when deciding on cases where there is no 'scientific consensus' regarding the plausibility of a proposed development,[81] with Benjamin J. Robertson further claiming this holds even in cases where the technologies described in a text are ones 'science tells us can never exist'.[82] Where developments like time travel sit on this spectrum is currently cause for much debate.

However, more recent scholarship has argued that Freedman, Bould and Miéville have simply conflated Suvin's 'cognition' with 'scientific plausibility'.[83] Rhys Williams provides a particularly compelling defence of Suvin's original conception, noting that any attempt to replace cognition with 'a voice that creates the "effect" of such cognition' is misguided, as this merely replaces Suvin's valuable principle of difference with the 'literary technique of verisimilitude'.[84] When considering that the very point behind the Brechtian *Verfremdungseffekt* was to remind the audience that what was being shown was *not* real, accusing Suvin of relying on cognitive validation from 'real science' seems especially peculiar. Perhaps the most damning account of Freedman's supposed point of difference from Suvin's definition comes from Freedman himself though, when he states that the 'readiest means of producing a cognition effect is precisely through cognition itself'.[85] As reproducing accurate science cannot logically be the defining characteristic of an estranged literature, Suvin's definition does not compel the field to reject Asimov's story as Freedman suggests. What matters is not whether Asimov's account of Mercury's rotation is strictly accurate, but that the rest of the story follows logically *if* it is – that is, the narrative relies on explanations of phenomena that are consistent with an internal, scientific logic that both avoids myth and magic and does not depend on external validation. Thus, the *appearance* of scientific plausibility was all that was ever at stake for Suvin, and as such, the supposed difference the 'cognition effect' is intended to make becomes, at least for Williams, functionally redundant. The best evidence supporting this is provided by Suvin's own extensive bibliographies of science fiction texts, which include many texts exploring scientific developments that had already been disproven at the time he was writing. His stated focus was instead on novelties that were 'directly continuous with (extrapolated from) *or at least analogous to* existing "scientific" cognitions', none of which would preclude tales like 'The Dying Night' from being selected and retained within the genre.[86] While Freedman's confessed goals are more focused on redefining science fiction exclusively within a Marxist frame and, most notably, retrospectively excluding what he refers to as the 'largely forgettable' American pulp tradition, his conflation of cognition with science fact undermines this endeavour.[87]

Another attempt to build on Suvin's definition is provided by Kathleen L. Spencer, who notes that while all fiction estranges, '[i]t is not the mere presence of estrangement, but the unusual degree of estrangement and the particular kinds of estranging devices it employs that distinguishes SF from other genres'.[88] Some typical examples include aliens, artificial intelligence, mutants and time travel, to name a few. Likewise, it is not the fact that a text is innovative that earns it a place in the genre, but rather that its central innovation, the *novum*, is totalizing – the narrative simply cannot be supported without it.[89] The *novum* is the difference that separates the real world from the science-fictional world and is what Suvin believes the science fiction classification hinges on.[90] Spencer's refinement can be used to deal with concerns regarding potentially *multi*-nova texts that are typically classified as science fiction.

While various innovations may co-exist in any one science-fictional text – for example, the Doctor from *Doctor Who* is both an alien *and* a space-time traveller – there is often a hierarchy that can be used to satisfy Suvin's demands for a novum that *dominates* the narrative. In the above instance, it could be argued that a human space-time traveller could support the narrative just as well as a Gallifreyan; in fact, for much of the series, the Doctor's alien heritage is almost incidental to the plot. The reciprocal cannot be said. Without the capacity to travel through time and space using the TARDIS,[91] the Doctor's story would need to be drastically changed. Drawing on the example of *The Island* (2005) again, that cloning, rather than ectogenesis, is the central *novum* of this text is clear, in that removing ectogenesis and having the clones gestated biologically would not materially damage the narrative (although, as discussed above, it would remove the potential for the repulsive images to do their visual work). What the clones are is far more important than how they came to be such. What is most interesting in this case, though, is not the potential conflict between dominant and subordinate *novum*-esque innovations, but rather how the association of the former (cloning) with the latter (ectogenesis) masks the irrelevance of artificial wombs for producing the abuses depicted. Even for scholars who challenge Suvin's single-novum premise, the fact that ectogenesis receives reflected blame through conflation with the far more vital narrative element of cloning is worth noting.

Importantly for a project focused on imagining better reproductive futures, Suvin includes utopian writing within his definition, claiming it as 'the *sociopolitical subgenre of science fiction*'.[92] Suvin considered utopian fiction particularly well suited to provide the social commentary he believed good science fiction should be capable of. According to Peter Fitting, utopian literature is typically that which is focused on exploring a fictional 'better' world and will oftentimes include a sort of 'blueprint' for how to get there.[93] While there are many different utopian forms, the 'classic' or 'blueprint' form is still considered the most prominent in the sub-genre.[94] Fátima Vieira provides a particularly useful definition of utopia in *The Cambridge Companion to Utopian Literature*:

> One of the main features of utopia as a literary genre is its relationship with reality. Utopists depart from the observation of the society they live in, note down the aspects that need to be changed and imagine a place where those problems have been solved … The fact that the utopian traveller departs from a real place, visits an imagined place and goes back home, situates utopia at the boundary between reality and fiction. This fiction is in fact important, not as an end in itself, but as a privileged means to convey a potentially subversive message … Anchored in a real society, the utopist puts forward plausible alternatives, basing them on meticulous analysis and evaluation of different cultures.[95]

The significance of this connection with the author's reality is considered in more detail later, but suffice it to say that, for Vieira and Suvin alike, the purpose of utopian literature is to educate readers and inform social change.

With its focus on alternatives to the social *status quo*, Alessa Johns notes utopian literature has 'always appeared useful to feminists', despite the fact women often '[fare] poorly in traditional blueprint utopias'.[96] She notes feminist utopias are less likely to provide socio-political blueprints than traditional utopias, being instead more 'process-oriented', focused on the necessary improvements in women's education and social (particularly reproductive) empowerment to achieve utopian ends.[97] This focus on process and activism qualifies many of these as 'critical utopias' according to Tom Moylan's definition, exemplified by such feminist examples as Joanna Russ' *The Female Man* (1975), Ursula K. Le Guin's *The Dispossessed* (1974) and Marge Piercy's *Woman on the Edge of Time* (1976).[98] In her chapter 'Being an Artificial Womb Machine-Human', Sümeyra Buran notes '[u]topian feminist sf reflects women's hopes concerning the freedom of their bodies in reproduction; it offers positive scenarios arising from the feminist adaptation of technology'.[99] However, she also relates that many feminist utopian writers 'speculate on single-gender worlds, particularly female-only utopias, and imagine female parthenogenesis reproduction', repeating Moylan's list above and adding Charlotte Perkins Gilman's *Herland* (1915), Mary E. Bradley Lane's *Mizora* (1890) and Shelley Singer's *The Demeter Flower* (1980), among others. Inclusion in Moylan's definition of 'critical utopia' requires both that the text gained a critical mass of followers and that it critiqued dominant ideologies in the author's reality.[100] For Brian Garvey, what is central to Moylan's classification was whether the utopia provided 'a visible means by which change can be effected'.[101] Early examples in the genre in which perfect societies were depicted as 'totalizing blueprints' without any guidance regarding how the necessary changes might be pursued were notably excluded.[102]

In a similar vein, Moylan later claimed that 'critical dystopias' promoted a utopian dream through depicting its negation.[103] Again, there was a focus on process rather than blueprint in this designation. Greg Claeys' definition of dystopian literature as that which 'portray[s] feasible negative visions of social and political development, cast principally in fictional form' disqualifies any text that relies on 'extraordinary or utterly unrealistic' departures from existing realities.[104] For Moylan, however, the most important element was whether the dystopia critically reflected on cultural systems, such as patriarchy and capitalism.

Relying on a Suvinian model for defining science fiction for a liberal feminist project is perhaps best understood by combining the practical need for clear genre guidelines with the political need for a theory sympathetic to the goal of producing a society that has achieved gender equality in reproductive labour. Milner describes Suvin's seminal text, *Metamorphoses of Science Fiction*, as being overly prescriptive in its genre definition and 'avowedly neo-Marxist',[105] and while both aspects have been cause for significant criticism since its publication, these are precisely the elements that make Suvin's definition well suited for the current task. As described above, most competing options lack firm inclusion criteria. Further, Suvin's clear inclusion of utopian literature as a sub-genre of science fiction is particularly valuable, as it allows for a diverse range of feminist utopias to be considered.[106] These include fictional societies in which emerging reproductive technologies can be critiqued, both at the individual and population levels. While Marxist and feminist concerns will not always align in such an analysis, there is nevertheless significant overlap, particularly when considering the potential for technology to replace exploitation of the socially disempowered.

Bioethics as a narrative genre

This book seeks to construct a pro-technological, feminist narrative of ectogenesis to challenge the dominant conservative narratives opposing this technology often found in bioethics scholarship. This first requires an exploration of how such narratives are typically constructed within this field of research and how such uses can be challenged. In the introduction to her collection, *Stories and Their Limits: Narrative Approaches to Bioethics*, Hilde Lindemann Nelson outlines 'five things to do with stories'.[107] The first is to read, listen to or view stories while paying close attention to the 'nuances and complexities' of the narratives, as a means of 'sharpening one's moral sensibilities'.[108] This involves allowing the author of the fiction to engage one's intellect and emotions, directing attention to particular aspects of the issues being discussed. Naming Martha Nussbaum as the best-known proponent of the theory that literature can develop 'the moral emotions', Nelson goes on to state:

> Nussbaum is quick to point out that the literary imagination will not always prevail against deep prejudices, but the proper response to this failure, she argues, is not to repudiate the imagination but to cultivate it more consistently and humanely.[109]

In 'Literature and the Moral Imagination', Nussbaum claims that 'moral vision finds in novels its most appropriate articulation' and that some literary texts are 'irreplaceably, works of moral philosophy'.[110] For Nussbaum, moral communication in literature is made possible through engagement with the 'emotional and imaginative richness' of the characters' 'moral efforts'.[111] Both of these authors argue that literature can have great educational impact, particularly with regard to helping readers empathize with people suffering disadvantages they are not themselves familiar with.[112] This may be done, for example, through depicting relatable characters and sharing their intimate struggles against racism, sexism, homophobia or other systematic discrimination. In the case of science fiction narratives, it opens up the possibility of exploring disadvantages either inflicted or relieved by future technologies.

Continuing with Nelson's approaches to using narratives in bioethics, the second method involves *telling* stories – choosing to share particular elements of one's personal experiences 'in the light of relevant moral ideas'.[113] In this way, moral decisions can be made in the present by considering past actions and weaving together a personal narrative that promotes the actualization of moral goals and identity in the future. Nelson's third approach is to *compare* stories to search for moral guidance, noting Albert Jonsen and Stephen Toulmin's practice of establishing 'paradigm cases' in which 'moral maxims and principles' are exemplified, such that like cases can then be reasoned through by analogy to this example.[114] The fourth approach is engaging in literary analysis and hermeneutics, searching for moral meaning in texts and reflecting on the ethical issues depicted in the relationships between individuals and social institutions. Finally, Nelson claims bioethicists can *invoke* stories 'to make or illustrate a moral point', with many using cautionary tales to highlight some moral danger.[115]

All five of the methods outlined above could be applied to investigating the role of science fiction in bioethics scholarship on ectogenesis, but this section particularly focuses on the use of stories to develop moral emotions and illustrate moral points. Later chapters also use literary analysis to explore the representation of ectogenesis in science fiction, tying this to various bioethical arguments regarding the technology. Such tools are suitable for analysing not only the representation of ectogenesis in fictional narratives but also those found within bioethics scholarship. As such, it is important to consider how utopian and dystopian cautionary tales are used in bioethical debates regarding emerging reproductive technologies, with such examples forming literary cases within the 'genre' of bioethics scholarship.

For Tod Chambers, the case studies that permeate bioethical discussion are themselves a narrative genre, opening up the possibility for narrative criticism to play a pivotal role in bioethics.[116] He notes that, like other genres, the field of bioethics has its own folkloric shorthand, for example, 'ethicists do not have to retell an entire story but can simply say "Dax" ' when wishing to discuss theories of patient autonomy, in reference to the famous case of Dax Cowart.[117] However, he claims that bioethicists often try to mask the significance of narrative stories to their craft by insisting the case studies they use are 'real', rather than fictional.[118] The tellers of these stories admit to them being anonymized and sometimes adapted to make them fit a certain argument better, but the core events, they claim, are based on real life. The prefaces of various bioethics textbooks are provided as evidence that bioethicists want readers to respond to their cases as if they are objective facts, with many stressing that the cases contained in their volume are based on actual events.[119] K. Danner Clouser claims this is one of the differences between the use of cases in moral philosophy compared with bioethics: moral philosophy uses fictional cases contrived to *illustrate* theories, whereas bioethicists use so-called 'real' cases in order to *test* ethical theories.[120] However, Chambers argues that if readers cannot tell the difference between a real and imaginary case without the aid of a preface, this indicates both types of narrative can achieve the same function and can be accepted as legitimate data for ethical consideration:

> The dichotomy that I have been interested in attacking has not been that there is no real difference between a real case and a fictional one – a difference between unconstructed and constructed cases – but that this difference in the end does not matter. Real people and real events must be turned into representations when they are transformed into narratives.[121]

Since all bioethics cases are thus narrativized, the rules of narrative analysis apply when taking a moral position, including consideration of whose points of view are being displayed in the case and the impact of narrative voice on the representation of salient moral issues. This also indicates that where 'real' cases are not possible, as in the case of speculative technologies, fictional cases provide a valuable substitute.

In response to Chambers' argument, James F. Childress accepts that bioethics cases are narratives, or at the very least 'mini-narratives' involving characters, plots and actions.[122] While disagreeing with some of Chambers' conclusions, Childress concedes that the tellers of bioethics cases (narrators) do have an ethical obligation to consider the narrative elements of their stories, including the use of language, metaphors and analogies, in order to ensure balanced representation.[123] The use of science-fictional references in bioethical debate often violates this obligation though, exploiting the ability of fictional narratives to stimulate the moral imagination without providing balanced analysis. According to James S. Terry and Peter C. Williams, moral sensitivity and empathy can be learned through fictional narratives, since they provide a 'vicarious experience' of ethical dilemmas or health events the person encountering the narrative may never have experienced in the real world.[124] As such, it is important to note which characters in a narrative are positioned sympathetically, which have agency in the plot of the story, and how the consequences of ethical decisions are portrayed.

Valentina Adami advocates for the use of the 'bioethics-in-literature' approach to investigating bioethical issues through the lens of literary fiction, allowing for a 'richly rendered and vividly presented' alternative to the dull, clinical case studies often used in discourse.[125] Like Tsitas, she claims that literary representations of bioethical issues help us see cases as 'embedded in specific human contexts and to understand the powerful emotions and intricate interpersonal dynamics that lie behind a bioethical case'.[126] However, as will be demonstrated in the following chapter, while science-fictional representations of ectogenesis are certainly 'richly rendered', when it comes to developing moral emotion or illustrating bioethical arguments, the overall pattern is negative. As a genre typically believed to open up imaginative possibilities, the techno-conservatism of many science fiction narratives when it comes to emerging reproductive technologies warrants careful consideration. Furthermore, where positive examples do exist in the genre, these are typically missing from bioethical debate. This is possibly due to the closer relationship the pragmatic manifestos of the future found within bioethical scholarship have with the blueprint form of utopian science fiction, a form less likely to be feminist. Even the typical practice of using thought experiments in bioethical discussion, where variables have been artificially limited to distil a single ethical dilemma, seems aimed at preventing a more open, process-based perspective. As will be explored in the next chapter, this often prevents the realization of science fiction's potential for bioethics in discussing methods of promoting sexual equality in human reproduction.

3

Science fiction engaging with bioethics

This chapter explores the representation of ectogenesis in science fiction and popular culture, paying particular attention to the bioethical issues these texts illustrate. Using several textual examples, common narrative tropes within science fiction literature and film regarding this emerging technology will be explored. It is not within the scope of this book to consider all the representations of ectogenesis to be found in science fiction; however, considering some of the recurrent themes and motifs associated with this emerging technology will illustrate some of the ways fiction authors engage with bioethical issues in their works. The next chapter will then explore the reciprocal relationship in which bioethicists use science-fictional references in debate.

The mad scientist 'Playing God'

As one of the key scientists involved in the first successful IVF birth, Robert Edwards received a lot of criticism for supposedly overstepping nature's bounds. In his book, *Life Before Birth*, Edwards recounts how the media vilified him for his work, leading to his barrister actioning six libel lawsuits for false claims, including allegedly concealing experimental results and advocating for human reproductive cloning.[1] Edwards notes that at the heart of these criticisms were 'undeniably genuine fears – of ectogenesis, animal uterine hosts, man/animal hybrids' and the fact that at the time there were no guidelines for scientists regarding what research in the area was ethically acceptable.[2] However, he also claims that: 'Somewhere, often unrecognised at the backs of people's minds, the picture lingers of the embryologist as a mad scientist, busily cloning monsters'.[3] Where did this lingering picture arise? One source of the 'mad scientist' motif is certainly the realm of science fiction and can be traced back to what some argue is the first novel of the genre, Mary Shelley's *Frankenstein*

(1818).[4] As noted in Chapter 1, the scientist responsible for the first IVF pregnancy in rabbits was also labelled Dr Frankenstein as a direct reference to the quintessential hubristic scientist, whose attempt to usurp God's role as the giver of life turned to disaster with the creation of a murderous and grotesque monster. In response to criticisms regarding his involvement in developing IVF, Edwards' partner Patrick Steptoe also famously declared: 'I am not a wizard or a Frankenstein'.[5]

There are many science-fictional texts that contain a mad or unscrupulous scientist experimenting with ectogenesis, often with no supervision or legal oversight. The doctor responsible for growing human clones using artificial wombs in the film *The Island* (2005) is depicted as being highly unstable, with colleagues saying he has a 'god complex'.[6] The creation of clones that can 'walk, talk and feel' is illegal in this fictional society; however, lax enforcement of these laws has allowed the doctor to build an entire community of fully conscious clones whose mental development is deliberately stunted to keep them compliant.[7] Similarly, the CEO of Replacement Technologies and main antagonist of *The 6th Day* (2000), Michael Drucker, uses ectogenesis to illegally grow human clones so that he can obsessively chase the goal of immortality. Drucker's classic villain speech to the film's protagonist, the clone of Adam Gibson, betrays his megalomaniacal belief that his 'higher purpose' is to achieve god-like power over death:

Drucker: In two years, three tops, I will control enough votes to get the laws changed. And then we won't have to lose our best people. We won't have to lose our Mozarts. We won't have to lose our Martin Luther Kings. We will finally be able to conquer death. *We will finally be able to conquer death!*

Gibson: And who gets to decide who lives and who dies, you?

Drucker: You have a better idea?

Gibson: Yeah. What about God?

Drucker: You're one of those. I suppose you think science is inherently evil.

Gibson: No. I don't think science is inherently evil. But I think you are.

Drucker: If you believe that God created man in his own image, then you also believe that God gave man the power to understand evolution, to exploit science, to manipulate the genetic code. To do exactly what I'm doing. I'm just taking over where God left off.[8]

With reference to narrative point of view (or focalization), it is noteworthy that the 'victims' in both of the above films are the ectogenetically grown clones whose perspective the audience follows throughout. Focalization will be discussed further in the final chapter, but for now, it is important to consider how presenting these characters as innocent victims necessarily implicates the medical staff and corporations responsible for developing and using the technology that created them. These characters, like Drucker above, are seen to be evil, even when their ultimate goals may be saving human lives. Similarly, in *The Island*, most of the childlike clones are created to provide autologous organs for transplant for paying customers, in what can be viewed as an extreme extension of the 'saviour sibling' practice in which parents use IVF to select embryos to implant that will be able to donate compatible tissue to an existing child with a medical condition. What makes *The Island* particularly horrifying is that the clones are usually terminated after harvesting, and these scenes are shot in a way that highlights the vulnerability of the clones, as they are both cognitively and physically restrained such that they cannot defend themselves. The clones end their lives as they began them, with bodily fluids gushing to the floor and skin pierced by a surgeon's scalpel, as with their violent 'deliveries' from their ectogenesis pods. Nevertheless, scientists in the film claim their research is justifiable, as it will one day lead to cures for conditions like leukaemia.[9] Like Drucker, these scientists excuse their immoral treatment of human clones by appealing to a classical utilitarian argument that they have a 'higher purpose' to support the greatest good for the greatest number.

The significance of these two textual examples is that they both support the idea that scientists cannot be trusted and that regulations restricting embryo experimentation are insufficient protection against misuse. They also perpetuate the techno-determinist view that if something *can* be done, it inevitably *will* be done, irrespective of legal and ethical obstacles, and society will be forced to adapt to whatever changes technology demands.[10] When these fears combine, they produce just one solution to the perceived threat of emerging biotechnologies – prevent them from coming into existence in the first place. By this logic, even if some scientists wanted to pursue ectogenesis for morally praiseworthy reasons – such as saving the lives of women who might otherwise die in childbirth – their research would *inevitably* be corrupted by others intent on pursuing unethical goals and thus should be prohibited.

This argument shares common ground with the traditional 'slippery slope' objection to assisted reproductive technologies, which Kieran Tranter claims considers everything from artificial insemination and IVF to embryo transfer and surrogacy as dangerous steps toward ectogenesis and human cloning.[11] John Mendeloff argues that the purpose of the slippery slope argument is to encourage policymakers and ethics committees to consider the future 'ethical costs' of their decisions in the present.[12] He continues by exploring the implication that reasons used for granting permission for research now will 'justify *in advance* future decisions that may be much more troubling'.[13] A relevant example might be the decision that women who have lost their uterus to cancer should be allowed to reproduce using ectogenesis, since they cannot achieve their goal of producing offspring without some recourse to assisted reproduction. Proponents of the slippery slope argument might argue this would lay the foundation for future parents to use ectogenesis to achieve other reproductive goals not naturally possible, such as human augmentation. However, the argument is not just used on one side of the techno-science debate. Leon Kass notes that those opposing placing limits on scientific development also use the 'much maligned slippery-slope argument', claiming that such restrictions would do 'great harm to scientific freedom'.[14] For both sides, the risks of allowing science and scientists to run amok are concerning, but their solutions differ from banning research to tolerating some harm as inevitable while still reaping the benefits of new technologies. For this book, the slippery slope argument represents one of the weaker objections to ectogenesis, especially when considering that historically, similar fears associated with reproductive technologies, such as IVF, turned out to be misguided. For example, despite the concerns Edwards noted above, the widespread uptake of IVF did not lead to the creation of animal-human hybrids.

Using Shelley's *Frankenstein* and Aldous Huxley's *Brave New World* as key examples, Lewis Wolpert claims: 'One will search with very little success for a novel in which scientists come out well'.[15] In her article, 'From Alchemy to Artificial Intelligence', Roslynn Haynes goes further to identify seven recurring stereotypes of scientists appearing in Western literature and film, displaying various characteristics of evil, noble heroism, foolishness, adventurousness, danger and helplessness. However, she claims there is a 'master narrative of the scientist' to be found among these stereotypes: 'the mad, bad, dangerous scientist, unscrupulous in the exercise of power'.[16] Haynes notes this stereotype provides 'a convenient shorthand' for writers and filmmakers when discussing scientists and scientific advancements, but that it oversimplifies the issues at stake, leading to confusion and disempowerment for an audience already fearing 'the power and change that science entails'.[17] The rhetorical power of associating emerging biotechnologies with caricatures of irresponsible scientists and doctors resides partly in the familiarity many readers and viewers have with the 'mad scientist' motif and partly in existing concerns about the potential for new technologies to disrupt socio-cultural equilibrium. Scepticism regarding the appropriate limitations to place on scientific and technological interventions into human reproduction can be explored effectively through science-fictional representations of future societies. However, when the creators and users of these technologies are overwhelmingly depicted as tragically insane, hopelessly naïve or dastardly evil, the opportunity for a serious discussion of the impact of emerging technologies on real-world societies is likely lost. Even purely allegorical readings of such texts are likely to buckle under the weight of such crude caricatures.

The message of films like *The Island* and *The 6th Day* is clear – if given the opportunity, the 'mad scientist' will develop ectogenesis for nefarious purposes, such as mass-market human cloning. They further imply that promoting ectogenesis research would open the floodgates for many other technological interventions into human reproduction. That human cloning could be achieved in the absence of ectogenesis is not considered by either text, as much of the visual horror relies on the viewer witnessing cloning that is externalized and produced on a large scale. This will be discussed in more detail with regard to the human farming trope in science fiction, but suffice it to say that ectogenesis is not necessary to produce the horrors of *The Island* or *The 6th Day* – but in both cases, it is used because it is visually disturbing in the context of these narratives. Ectogenesis is often presented as if it will provide a unique means to achieve an undesirable outcome – in this case, mass market cloning – despite only being peripherally connected to this end result.

Animal-human hybrids

The themes explored above are pushed even further in the film *Splice* (2009), which is more explicit in its discussion of 'mad scientists', again relying on comparisons to Dr Frankenstein to illustrate how the scientists responsible for growing an animal-human hybrid in the lab have pushed the boundaries of science too far.[18] In this film, Clive and Elsa, a couple working in genetics research, create a cross-species chimera through ectogenesis. Unbeknownst to Clive, Elsa adds her own genetic material into the mix. Despite never wanting to be pregnant or have children, Elsa forms a strong maternal bond to the resultant creature, Dren, with the couple smuggling her out of the lab and adopting her as their child. Ethical issues that are brought up in the film include how an animal-human hybrid should be treated, how much responsibility scientists should take for what they create in the lab and whether it can ever be morally acceptable to suppress research that has the potential to save people's lives. Specifically, characters suggest moral outrage is standing in the way of beneficial genetics research that could treat conditions like cancer. While the audience is initially positioned to sympathize with Dren, whose cherub-like appearance belies a hidden, predatory nature, by the end of the film, it is clear that the violation of nature has had serious consequences. In what can only be described as a disturbingly regressive and Oedipal vision of gender roles, as a female, Dren seduces her father figure, but when she later transitions into a male, proceeds to murder Clive before raping Elsa. The superfluous nature of the ectogenesis chamber to achieve the animal-human hybrid in the first place is then brought into stark contrast when the film ends with a pregnant Elsa carrying Dren's offspring. Again, the technology appears to have been used for visual effect, with the insertion of the human DNA into the chamber being one of the most dramatic and threatening moments of the film.

As a science fiction horror film, *Splice* succeeds in its primary goal of eliciting a sense of terror. With most of the action taking place in either a cold, sterile lab or a creepy, dark and secluded barnyard, the audience's feelings of alienation are heightened. The constant threat of discovery adds tension to the narrative, but the major lesson to be learnt is that these scientists should have been supervised more closely. They even say themselves that they should not have 'changed the rules' and started creating 'monsters'.[19] As Edwards' quote from the previous section demonstrates, fears that reproductive scientists were going to transgress the animal/human divide were responsible for much of the initial concern regarding IVF. Philip J. Nickel claims that horror can be fuelled both by tapping into realistic fears and anxieties, such as the risk of 'technology gone amok', and by invoking terrifying monsters that may, or may not, symbolize something horrific in the real world.[20] *Splice* successfully manages to combine these horror-provoking elements into one animal-human hybrid, with the horror being reinforced through association with real social anxieties about genetic manipulation. While Carroll claims that science fiction scholars often consider monsters to 'play second fiddle to the imagination of alternative technologies' within the genre,[21] in the case of Dren, the monster has not only been created by gene hybridization technology, it actually *becomes* the technology. In this way, the text also fits within the growing sub-genre of medical technology horror, which Carroll claims preys on 'culture's prevailing fears', representing transgressions from the norm.[22] In this case, the transgression involves violating the clear delineation of human and non-human.

As a real-world example, Australia's National Health and Medical Research Council (NHMRC) still considers any research involving the transfer of living cells from one species to another (xenotransplantation) to pose 'unique public health and ethical challenges that warrant special consideration'.[23] Concerns regarding xenotransplantation are focused predominantly on the risk of transmitting diseases from animal species into the human population, rather than the creation of unnatural monsters in the lab, though. Nevertheless, it is this potentiality that fascinates fiction writers, with various episodes of the long-running science fiction classic television series, *The X-files* (1993–2016), also focused on the creation of *alien*-human hybrids. Some of these creations appear to have been grown ectogenetically, while others were gestated inside of comatose female patients.[24]

From a bioethical perspective, the real issue being dramatized in these stories of hybrids is what rights should be afforded to new organisms, particularly if they contain human DNA. While in most cases ectogenesis is not strictly necessary to conduct the experiments yielding such creatures, as many could be naturally gestated inside human wombs, the use of this technology allows the audience to visualize the merging of animal and human characteristics in a way that challenges anthropocentric assumptions about human uniqueness. The significance of this is underscored by the fact that rights are often bestowed on animals according to the degree to which they approximate human behaviours, and the human foetus is typically afforded increasing levels of legal protection relative to its closeness to independent human function. In *Splice*, Dren is treated like a child because she *looks* like a child, demonstrating the power of representation on how an organism is treated.

At present, it is not just hybrids that represent a potentially new moral and legal quagmire but artificially gestated human infants as well. As all children heretofore have been born 'of woman', Steiger notes that the acquisition of full legal personhood has usually coincided with 'complete extrusion of a newborn baby from the mother's body'.[25] He notes such a definition could not be consistently applied to foetuses developed using ectogenesis technology, as they may never have been housed in, nor extracted from, another's body. According to Bayne and Kolers, by some legal and social definitions of parenthood, such children would also be considered orphans.[26] So, while what might go into an ectogenesis chamber in the real world might differ substantially from the genetically engineered monsters of science fiction, what comes out still poses a challenge for lawyers and ethicists alike.

Genetic manipulation, human enhancement, and super soldiers

More common than creating hybrids is science fiction's propensity to genetically engineer 'superior' humans. As seen in the examples discussed above, ectogenesis is often incidental to what Suvin would consider the true 'novum'[27] of these science fiction texts. However, for the children's science fiction television series, *Kyle XY* (2006–2009), ectogenesis represents the central method of achieving the genetic and biological manipulation of a human 'super soldier'.[28] This is a particularly interesting text, not only because of the centrality of ectogenesis to the plot but also because, unlike similar super soldier narratives – for example, those focused on the Colonists in *The X-Files* or the Augments in *Star Trek* – *Kyle XY* depicts ectogenesis technology in a mostly positive light. The company responsible for artificially gestating the titular character until the age of sixteen certainly has sinister motives, but being gestated artificially is also seen to confer significant benefits to Kyle, including enhanced intelligence and physical strength. The creator of the artificial womb in the series, Adam Baylin, eventually reveals that his research was motivated by the loss of his own mother in childbirth and the desire to create an advanced civilization. Baylin designs a method of nourishing a developing foetus artificially that negates the need for an umbilical cord, and thus his creations noticeably lack a belly button.

In the real world, one of the major concerns about ectogenesis evidenced in bioethics scholarship is the potential for this technology to be used to create enhanced 'designer babies' through genetic engineering, selective implantation and scientific manipulation of the foetal growth environment. For *Kyle XY*, many of the enhancements Baylin achieves are a result of being able to extend the period of human gestation well beyond that which could be accommodated in a woman's body. This is also a feature of the human augmentation achieved for the In Vitroes of *Space: Above and Beyond* (1995–1996), who are likewise artificially gestated to adulthood and endowed with various genetic enhancements. This potential for ectogenesis to beneficially prolong gestation is also briefly addressed in Marge Piercy's *Woman on the Edge of Time* (1976), which will be discussed in further detail later in this chapter. With reference to those arguments focused on improving foetal outcomes through ectogenesis, Kyle makes an interesting case study for exploring how foetal manipulation and enhancement might actually play out. For example, despite enhancements intended to make him the perfect soldier, Kyle refuses to use his fighting skills in service of his creators.

His enhanced foreign language skills are also mostly wasted, as he chooses not to travel the world conducting secret missions, but rather to live the quiet life of a suburban teen attending high school. In this way, the manipulation of Kyle's genome and the circumstances surrounding his gestation fail to achieve their objective, with Kyle's personal autonomy remaining intact. Similarly, in bioethical discussions of the risk that genetic enhancement will diminish a child's 'right to an open future',[29] the role of personal preference and choice is often posited as a defence.

Arguments in favour of allowing ectogenesis to be used for eugenicist aims often rely on the idea of procreative beneficence, a theory put forward by Julian Savulescu that establishes a right *and duty* for parents to produce the best children possible.[30] This requires that when given the opportunity – through such technologies as IVF, pre-implantation genetic diagnosis (PGD) and, in the future, ectogenesis – parents ought to select the embryos and gestational methods expected to produce children with the best quality of life. Assuming the system was otherwise safe, the ability to avoid foetal complications, teratogenic exposures and birth trauma through using artificial, rather than biological, gestation would also make ectogenesis a desirable option for adherents of procreative beneficence.[31]

The obvious problem of determining which complement of genes or abilities is most likely to improve quality of life is not addressed directly in *Kyle XY*, but the assumption is that his acquired skills make him a superior soldier and human being. However, the issues around trying to breed better humans are dramatized well in Yevgeny Zamyatin's classic dystopia *We* (1924), in which only those considered 'eugenically fit' by the authoritarian Benefactor are allowed to breed.[32] In this text, the ramifications of a strict adherence to procreative beneficence and pursuit of eugenics include the One State taking complete control of sexual behaviour for the numbered citizens, mandating that all sexual partnerships be impersonal and allocated by the State. As such, the affair between the protagonist, D-503, and I-330, the woman he meets during the course of the narrative, is illegal, as is the request by D-503's sanctioned partner, O-90, that he impregnate her despite her failing the height requirements to be a mother.[33] Thus, the impact of pursuing human enhancement on personal relationships and sexual freedom is a central theme of this novel, whereas, as a show intended for children, the wider implications of Kyle's genetic modifications, non-sexual conception and motherless birth are mostly ignored, with focus remaining on his super abilities. Despite the radical disruption to traditional views of pregnancy depicted in the show, Kyle's adoptive mother is shown to be very traditional – the carer, cook and cleaner for her husband and children who sacrifices her career goals to support her family. It appears a positive representation of ectogenesis can only be supported if shown alongside a conservative view of family life and gender roles. Such a position is hardly rare in literature and film intended for children, with Karin Lesnik-Oberstein claiming that the dominant conservatism seen in children's entertainment is intended to train children to 'depend on authority' in the form of parents and law enforcement.[34] Due to his unconventional birth, Kyle must be socialized in a traditional family unit to provide appropriate authority figures to turn to for guidance and comfort. This fits with the general assumption, critiqued by many scholars, that texts for children should necessarily be pedagogical and aimed at promoting moral development within the narrow confines of the societal *status quo*.[35] Whether intentional or not, *Kyle XY* gives the impression that it is overcompensating for the one radical difference it has allowed through promoting a stereotypical, conservative image of the ideal nuclear family.

Human farming for resources

Connected to the super soldier trope is the idea of cultivating humans artificially for specified purposes. Kyle and the various other children Baylin creates were grown to be advanced human weapons, a goal also shared by Walter Bishop, the deranged scientist from the popular science fiction television series, *Fringe* (2008–2013), who experimented with ectogenesis as part of a secret government project focused on rapid maturation of a new human army.[36] As discussed earlier, *The Island* similarly involves 'farming' humans but in this instance for replacement body parts. Arguably, the most gripping example of the human farming trope in science fiction film, however, appears in *The Matrix* (1999). This film is also useful when considering the potential for ectogenesis to lead to the mass production of humans as a material resource. In this film, machines endowed with artificial intelligence have revolted against their human creators and now grow 'crops' of humans as a source of bio-electrical power. The humans are developed and sustained in pods, with their minds connected to a sophisticated artificial reality, so they remain unaware of their state of captivity. This mass production of humans as a means of meeting the machines' power needs is viewed as the grossest violation of human dignity. The following is an exchange between the protagonist, Neo, and the human resistance leader, Morpheus, who freed him from the Matrix:

> Morpheus: There are fields, Neo. Endless fields, where human beings are no longer born. We are grown. For the longest time, I wouldn't believe it. And then I saw the fields with my own eyes, watched them liquefy the dead so they could be fed intravenously to the living. And standing there, facing the pure horrifying precision, I came to realize the obviousness of the truth. What is the Matrix? Control. … As long as the Matrix exists the human race will never be free.[37]

The horrifying images of rows and rows of ectogenesis pods facing the newly released Neo in 'the real world' are a contrast to the neutral vision of late 1990s America depicted in the Matrix itself. This is particularly noteworthy since it is the artificial reality imprisoning the human population that is supposed to represent the true horror of the film.

In philosophical terms, *The Matrix* highlights Kantian concerns regarding using people as a 'mere means' to an end, in this case, power generation.[38] Were there any reciprocal benefits to the humans trapped in the Matrix, this could at least be seen as mutually advantageous exploitation, but as it is, the machines purely instrumentalize the people they enslave, demeaning their humanity and denying their intrinsic value. The machines could achieve their goal of collecting humans' bio-electricity through capturing adult humans and hooking them up to generators; however, instead they choose to grow humans from foetuses to adults, recycling their biological matter when they die. As such, they are not only *using* human lives for their own gain, they are *creating* them solely for this instrumental purpose.

As a bioethical case study, this distinction is important when considering the potential for ectogenesis to lead to greater commodification of children as 'products' their parents can 'commission'. Iina Hellsten claims that in public debates regarding new technologies, 'the consequences of overstepping the moral boundaries between human beings and mass products' are a central concern determining how the technology will be perceived and treated.[39] Some of these fears of commodification relate directly to the potential for ectogenesis to produce human beings *en masse*, an issue that is typically dramatized in science fiction by visual images of factory-like production lines or vast collections of pods displaying humans at various gestational stages of development.

Cloning

Similar to the concerns about the indignity of human farming are those connected to human reproductive cloning. In 1997, the United Nations Educational, Scientific and Cultural Organization (UNESCO) released the

Universal Declaration on the Human Genome and Human Rights, which claims that human reproductive cloning should not be permitted because it is 'contrary to human dignity'.[40] This general prohibition was recommended in spite of the Organization simultaneously decrying any attempt to reduce human beings to their genetic characteristics or engaging in genetic discrimination.[41] Faith Kabata and Donrich Thaldar note the significance of this Declaration claiming the human genome as 'common heritage of mankind', placing it in the same category as 'outer space, the moon and other celestial bodies, as well as the deep seabed'.[42] The Organization's opposition to human cloning still stands firm today.

As is clear from several of the above analyses, many examples of ectogenesis in science fiction texts also involve human cloning, thus conflating the ethical issues of one technology with another. The obvious case study to use regarding the impact of this fictional convergence is Huxley's dystopian classic, *Brave New World* (1932), a text that is frequently used and misused in bioethics scholarship. In an article for *USA Today*, Christiane Nüsslein-Volhard describes the future of reproduction as depicted in *Brave New World*:

> Huxley imagines a procedure by which embryos can be made to form buds, such that from one embryo several identical copies can develop. These cloned embryos then are to be raised in bottles that serve as a kind of artificial uterus. The realism of his story is buttressed by Huxley's detailed description of the physical and technical difficulties of the uterus machine. Most striking perhaps is his conjecture that the conditions under which the clones mature can be manipulated to program the desired attributes of these parentless beings.[43]

Nüsslein-Volhard notes that the most remarkable thing about the persistence of *Brave New World* in discussions of embryology is the fact that 'there are people who take Huxley's ideas as present or future truth rather than as the fiction that they are'.[44] Ball claims that only a 'lazy reading presents all this as a prescient feat of brilliant imagination', suggesting Huxley's 'political setting for ectogenetic anthropoeia has scant application to the twenty-first century'.[45] While holding genuine concerns about the ethical and social implications of ectogenesis, Ball argues that Huxleyan imagery and science-fictional concerns with 'gender annihilation, subhuman monsters and unnatural progeny' are hardly an appropriate framework within which to debate these.[46] Nevertheless, as will be demonstrated throughout the coming chapters, such a framework has become embedded within bioethics scholarship focused on ectogenesis. Huxley's dystopian future involves classical conditioning of ectogenetically grown clones that are genetically engineered to fulfil a pre-determined role in society. The production line mentality to mass reproduction is highlighted by the glorification of Fordism in the narrative, a reference to Henry Ford's assembly line production method for building cars. As with the human farming trope, the loss of human dignity involved in this mass reproduction is vividly displayed.

Peter Firchow considers *Brave New World* Huxley's 'most powerful rendering of the effects of science and technology' on human society, claiming it retains relevance to *any* discussion of the future of humanity over the 'next few centuries'.[47] Even a cursory review of bioethics and medical literature will find multiple references to this text when discussing numerous reproductive biotechnologies and other bioethical concerns. One example can be seen in D. S. Ferber's 2004 article, 'Miracle in Iowa', in which he searched for the novel's title in the Medline database, generating 200 positive results.[48] The same search twenty years later yields almost three times this number. However, the association of artificial gestation with the human cloning depicted in *Brave New World* is problematic, as it perpetuates the belief that the one will inevitably lead to the other. Dating back to 1983, a legal article written by George P. Smith II illustrates this belief well in a footnote in which he discusses ectogenesis, claiming: 'If human cloning were to succeed, ectogenesis would have to be perfected to a high degree'.[49] At the same time, bioethicist William A. W. Walters made a similar claim, suggesting ectogenesis would be necessary 'if the cloning of human beings was to go ahead enthusiastically in large numbers'.[50] This latter quote is more accurate, as just like in the case of Huxley's dystopia, ectogenesis is not *necessary* to produce human clones in the real world, but it might be practically *convenient* if the goal were to create clones at any great scale.

Ball argues that *Brave New World* is frequently misappropriated 'as if it was a work of futurology' rather than a 'bleak social satire of its times', claiming that one explanation for the pervasiveness of this text in discussions about emerging technologies is that it feeds 'myths we want to believe'.[51] However, Andrew Milner et al. argue that while science fiction should not be treated as futurology, it should 'ideally function as an adjunct to "futurology"', quoting George Turner's claim that the genre is in a unique position to serve as 'a useful tool for serious consideration, on the level of the non-specialist reader, of a future rushing on us at an unstoppable speed'.[52] While justifying some claims that science fiction authors should be more nuanced in their use of biotechnological innovations due to the potential to impact perceptions of emerging technologies, what is more important here is how bioethicists should engage with such texts. Often, the use of *Brave New World* in bioethical scholarship regarding ectogenesis feeds into the myth that this technology is somehow intrinsically linked with a threatening future of mass human cloning.

Biological pregnancy unavailable

A somewhat rarer use for ectogenesis in science fiction is as a substitute for natural gestation because women are not physically available to be pregnant. One example of this appears in the 1980s' *The Terminator* comic series produced by NOW Comics, in which ectogenesis chambers are created to take over the task of gestating the next generation of humans, so female soldiers do not need to leave the frontlines to give birth.[53] In their war against the Terminators, humanity cannot spare fighters but must be able to replenish their ranks of soldiers, so artificial gestation is considered a viable alternative that also avoids any physical debilitation the female soldiers might otherwise suffer during pregnancy. Although the women may consider this beneficial, their perspective is not included in the comic's narrative, and the intention of developing the technology was not to promote women's interests or sexual equality but to support the war effort. As this series is quite obscure, it is unlikely to appear in bioethics scholarship. Nevertheless, it is still interesting to consider on what grounds people suggest the development of ectogenesis can be reasonably justified. In this case, the necessity of war demands alternatives to physical gestation, with no regard for maternal or foetal interests. Similar uses also appear in more well-known science fiction, like Weber's *At All Costs* (2005) from the Honorverse series, where the protagonist, naval officer Honor Harrington, transfers her pregnancy to an artificial womb so as not to interfere with her deployment.[54]

Another example of this trope can be seen in Lois McMaster Bujold's *Ethan of Athos* (1986), part of the Vorkosigan Saga, in which an all-male planet uses ectogenesis to procreate in the absence of any women. The analysis of this story addresses one of the traditional feminist objections to ectogenesis – the argument that it would render women expendable, thereby leaving them vulnerable to 'femicide' by patriarchal powers. Like the other men of Athos, the story's protagonist, Dr Ethan Urquhart, is deeply suspicious and frightened of women, whom his religious community has taught him are immoral and depraved creatures. When he must travel off-world to purchase ovarian cultures to prevent population decline, Ethan encounters women like many other science fiction heroes may encounter an alien species. His description of them as 'uterine replicators with legs' demonstrates that within his culture, where ectogenesis has replaced biological gestation, women are considered superfluous.[55] This seems to support the belief that women's role in procreation is the single contribution to society that can save them from annihilation, harkening back to Corea's arguments mentioned in the Introduction. However, this neglects the various other roles women fulfil within modern society, many of which are highly prized even in cultures that are deeply patriarchal.

In terms of bioethical discussions, removing the *option* of natural gestation challenges assumptions about how procreation ought to occur in society. This ties into common arguments about reproductive biotechnologies and whether they should be available on demand or only in cases of 'medical necessity'. This has led to various discriminatory policies for prospective parents seeking to use assisted reproduction for social, rather than physiological, infertility, including in terms of public funding.[56] In both *The Terminator* comic and *Ethan of Athos*, ectogenesis is justified due to the threat of extinction without it. This justification is often also present in the next trope to be considered here, using artificial wombs to gestate a future human space colony.

Space colonization

Another reason ectogenesis may be used in a science-fictional world is to support off-world population growth for a human settlement. One recent example can be found in Guy Immega's *Super-Earth Mother: The AI that Engineered a Brave New World* (2023), in which a self-aware, artificial general intelligence known as 'Mother-9' takes humanity's genetic material and uses artificial wombs to gestate a colony of humans following the destruction of Earth. In the Prologue, Mother-9 claims there is 'no greater goal than colonizing the galaxy', noting that their purpose is to 'conceive and nurture humans on an exoplanet'.[57] This leads to the following conversation with their creator, the wealthy and narcissistic Walcott:

> 'We'll all be dead by then. Civilization won't last that long'.
>
> I tried to reassure him. 'That's why I'm going to a new world. When I arrive, I'll synthesize human life, chromosome by chromosome. Baby by baby, I'll build a breeding population. Our exocolony will ensure the survival of the human race beyond Earth. It'll be a planned paradise, a new utopia, the Walcott legacy'.[58]

Walcott's legacy is functionally a Noah's Ark project, aimed at achieving species preservation through the selection of supposedly superior humans (or in this case, their DNA). The issue of embryo space colonization using ectogenesis has featured several times in recent space ethics scholarship,[59] with some authors even specifically noting the role artificial intelligence may play in this project.[60] However, the above quote also demonstrates two related ethical concerns for off-world migration more broadly: how might a sample of humans be selected for evacuation should Earth become uninhabitable; and how can an off-world colony be created without sacrificing reproductive liberty for the settlers.[61] In the first instance, classical lifeboat ethics suggests the greater good is served by saving some humans even at the expense of others and even when principles of equity and justice are necessarily violated in the selection process. In its original, and rather distasteful formulation, lifeboat ethics was used by eugenicist Garrett Hardin to oppose the provision of humanitarian aid to the disadvantaged.[62] The views of the character Walcott would fit well with Hardin's supporters. In the second instance, if only physiologically fertile candidates are considered for off-world exploration, this represents both discrimination against equally qualified but physically or socially infertile peers and a source of undue pressure to procreate among those selected. Mother-9's goal to create a 'breeding population' can thus be seen to undermine reproductive autonomy for the resultant colonists.

An older science fiction, *The Dragons of Heorot* (1995) – a.k.a. *Beowulf's Children* (1996) – further considers the potential for ectogenesis to circumvent any genetic damage space-faring adults may suffer due to cosmic radiation, using reproductive technologies to protect the viability of an off-world population both through artificial gestation and genetic engineering.[63] Due to a number of socio-biological complications, the result is not the utopian society desired though. In the real world, protecting the developing foetus against space hazards is one of the main justifications put forward for pursuing ectogenesis for space exploration. While avoiding teratogens would be easier for any *ex utero* pregnancy, when considering the harsh environment of space, the benefit of being able to separate the foetus from its progenitor becomes more obvious.[64]

The treatment of ectogenesis in Immega's novel is unique as the text explicitly mentions that the artificial wombs involve 'full ectogenesis' and are not 'just "biobags" for a fetus removed from the natural mother', indicating familiarity with both the state of the science of ectogenesis and the ethical debates regarding the difference between full and partial ectogenesis.[65] The depiction also contains elements of several of the tropes listed above, including using artificial gestation to produce clones and hybrids and engage in human augmentation through genetic modification. In the first chapter of the story, the foetus being 'brewed' in a prototype artificial womb is described as 'the first GMO human with synthesized DNA ... a chimera, a mix of many people. It's called pantropy – modifying humans to live in new environments'.[66] The developing foetus is dubbed 'Franky, spelled with a Y for his male chromosome', with the character responsible for the trial insisting the child won't be a 'Frankenstein monster' though, because errors in their genome have been corrected using CRISPR gene editing technology.[67] As with various other examples considered in this chapter, neither the genetic engineering nor the chimerism achieved for Franky depend on artificial gestation. That the Y chromosome used to create Franky was 'copied from a public library' is relevant for the next issue to be discussed here, non-consensual genetic parenthood.[68]

Involuntary genetic parenthood

In an article for the *Southern California Law Review*, I. Glenn Cohen discusses the pros and cons of establishing a legal right *not* to be a genetic parent. Recognizing that current protections for women against interference with the continuation of their pregnancies, or terminations of the same, rely on appeals to the right to bodily integrity that do not apply in the context of becoming a genetic (but not gestational) parent, Cohen continues by considering whether there can plausibly be a right to control one's biological material after it is separated from one's body.[69] Claiming that the deliberate use of a person's sperm or ova against their will for procreative purposes is the 'archetypal instance of treating another as a mere means to our own end', Cohen notes that there are many individuals who are genetic parents who did not consent to this situation.[70] This is most commonly experienced by men, who in most genuine democracies can neither force a woman to continue nor terminate a pregnancy, regardless of any genetic relationship he has with the resultant offspring. In a lot of cases, men may remain unaware that they have even become genetic parents. Ectogenesis represents a method by which women could also become genetic parents without their knowledge or consent. While this is already theoretically possible if IVF embryos were to be misappropriated and implanted in a surrogate without the genetic mother's knowledge, there are various other possibilities for involuntary genetic parenthood facilitated by ectogenesis that are explored in several science-fictional texts, particularly those associated with the superhero sub-genre.

Offspring of superheroes created artificially in the laboratory include Nate Grey from the *X-man* comic book series (1995–2001), genetic son of Jean Grey (Phoenix) and Scott Summers (Cyclops); Damian Wayne from the 'Batman and

Son' comic book story arc (2006) within the *Batman* series (1940–), genetic son of Bruce Wayne (Batman) and Talia al Ghul; and Connor Kent, a.k.a. Superboy, originally from *The Adventures of Superman* (1993) and later from the D.C. New 52 *Superboy* (2011–2014) comic, genetically derived from Superman (either as a clone of him or his future son, Jon Lane Kent), and often also his arch nemesis, Lex Luthor.[71] In each of these cases, the intention of combining the relevant genetic samples and gestating the foetus artificially is to cultivate multiple superhero powers. A secondary objective is often to complicate the lives of the heroes in the series, who are typically unaware for some time that they have become genetic parents, sometimes sharing this role with one of their enemies. That it is not necessary for either genetic parent to physically interact with the other or the resultant child at any stage in its development highlights the complete separation of sexual activity and gestational labour from procreation that ectogenesis allows. For Farquhar, reproductive technologies that can lead to such a separation challenge 'the naturalized assumption that reproduction is heterosexual and heterosocial', leading to the radical division of maternity into 'genetic-ovarian, gestational-uterine, and legal-social dimensions'.[72] However, ectogenesis takes things one step further by eliminating the gestational-uterine dimension altogether. As with most reproductive technologies, any phallocentric assumptions regarding traditional reproductive sex are also abandoned, as male sexual activity at any stage in the process is no longer required to achieve pregnancy.[73] This is especially the case when the male genetic material is harvested from somatic cells, such as skin cells, rather than sperm.[74]

Unlike in the cases of involuntary genetic parenthood currently possible, ectogenesis provides the means for a male scientist – like Mr Sinister from *X-man*, for example – to create a child without *any* female having knowledge of it, not even a surrogate. This would seem to meet Rosi Braidotti's definition of the alchemist's goal, the ability to create life without the need for women or the 'imperfection of the natural course of events' that occur in the dark and unknown uterus.[75] In 'Evolution's Pregnant Pause', medical ethicist, Joseph Fletcher, provides evidence to support Braidotti's claim, going as far as claiming the natural womb is a 'hazardous environment' for foetal development and that ectogenesis would be preferable because it allows children to be 'watched and protected as much as possible'.[76] For Braidotti, '[o]n the imaginary level, therefore, the test-tube babies of today mark the long-term triumph of the alchemists' dream of dominating nature through their self-inseminating, masturbatory practices'.[77] Feminist critics including O'Brien and Adrienne Rich have explained this desire by claiming men are jealous of the unique power over creating life that women possess, leading them to impose restrictions on women's behaviour.[78] Braidotti notes that this has also led to various sperm-centred models of human reproduction throughout history, including the Aristotelian view of women as 'passive receptacles' for men's life-giving seed.[79] In her book, *Pregnant Men*, Ruth Colker suggests that men are still 'socialized to overvalue their sperm, because their sperm is their only connection to reproduction'.[80] Such elevation of the genetic aspect of parenthood over the gestational or social is also clear through the treatment of characters like Damian Wayne. He is considered Bruce Wayne's son by virtue of this genetic tie alone, eventually also appropriating the mantle of Batman's sidekick, Robin. This prioritizing of genetic relationships and, in particular, genetic paternity is exactly what Raymond challenges with her concept of 'ejaculatory fatherhood', in which she dismisses equal or superior parental claims based on patrilineal relationships.[81]

Sexual equality

The final reason for using ectogenesis in science fiction is the one that is most central to this book, but possibly least represented in the genre. It is also the fictional representation most lacking in bioethics scholarship that engages with science fiction, that is, the use of this emerging biotechnology to promote sexual equality in human reproduction. In the utopian futures imagined by feminist writers Firestone and Piercy, the unequal distribution of the burdens of reproduction across the sexes is redressed through ectogenesis. As Steiger notes, some consider ectogenesis a necessary condition for achieving sexual equality due to the belief that 'because childcare responsibility has always been biologically linked to women, true equality will only occur once both sexes have an identical role in reproduction'.[82] In reference to Piercy's vision of the future in *Woman on the Edge of Time* (1976), Alice Adam further claims: 'Even those who are disturbed by the prospect of extrauterine reproduction often find the resulting utopian society appealing'.[83] At the core of Piercy's utopia is the belief that human reproduction is fundamentally a source of oppression for women.[84] As such, in an idealized version of the future, physiological gestation is replaced with artificial gestation in order to liberate women from this oppression. This is seen to yield benefits for society as a whole and women in particular, in addition to allowing for a degree of foetal enhancement through prolonged gestation and scientific manipulation. Kathy Rudy notes:

> While Piercy's utopia may be a far cry from the world we experience today, I believe that the development and practice of ectogenesis would help us move closer to such a dream. … With the help of *Woman on the Edge of Time*, we can see the possibility that ectogenesis might help eliminate the gap between the genders and render some modes of sexism obsolete. In a world in which babies are grown in tanks or bottles, there would be no need for surrogate mothers … the implantation of an invitro fertilization into a woman's body would be rendered unnecessary … and the technological focus on the fetus might never exploit another human being.[85]

Commonly considered as one of only a handful of science fiction texts in which ectogenesis is painted in a positive light,[86] *Woman on the Edge of Time* provides a literary counterargument to the objections highlighted in many of the texts discussed above. While in the minority, depictions of ectogenesis as a potentially equalizing technology are valuable in bioethical debate. Narratologically, it is significant that Piercy's protagonist is a woman who has been victimized by biological gestation, providing a direct contrast to Adam Gibson from *The 6th Day* and the clones from *The Island*, whose misfortunes relate back to their artificial gestation.

When considering the potential for ectogenesis to reduce both male and female contributions to reproduction to 'gamete provision', Farquhar claims this 'seems to be neither an unequivocal loss nor gain'.[87] However, she does concede that women's bodies are the ones 'put at risk, pained, and worked on (and up) because of the vicissitudes of female reproductive biology',[88] which would seem to support the claim that some women would consider artificial gestation a desirable alternative. Thus, it is easy to see why feminist science fiction authors in particular took an interest in ectogenesis as a plot device, exploring both the pros and cons of developing this technology. Ball notes that in many cases, these writers anticipated the discussions that would later occur between scientists and social critics regarding the potential impacts of ectogenesis.[89] Vera Brittain's *Halcyon, or The Future of Monogamy* (1929), is a particularly interesting case study, in which the development of ectogenesis was necessary to highlight the inequalities women faced in reproduction, only to be rejected as an inferior method of gestation necessitating dramatically improved conditions for pregnancy and childbirth in order to entice women back to this method. Even though Brittain was opposed to ectogenesis in her story – except as a last resort for otherwise unsafe pregnancies – it still served a vital function in achieving her feminist objective of greater sexual equality.[90] As such, Squier notes ectogenesis represented for Brittain 'a temporary stage in the process of shaping pregnancy along feminist lines'.[91] The relevant point is that before the development of a viable alternative, women had insufficient negotiating power to demand improvements to their current situation. This more moderate position provides a valuable comparison to Firestone and Piercy.

A more recent example where ectogenesis is used in science fiction to pursue certain liberal feminist objectives is *The Pod Generation* (2023). In this narrative, couples have the option of gestating their offspring in egg-shaped pods, with some companies even contributing to the substantial cost as a corporate strategy to 'retain the best and brightest women' in their workforce.[92] The arguments in favour of the technology echo many of the feminist arguments discussed in previous chapters, with the Pegazus company's Womb Center advertising claiming the pods 'help solve childbirth and empower women, and men of course'.[93] Customers seen accessing the technology include heterosexual and same-sex couples and singletons, including women using their own stem cells to fertilize their ova, bypassing the need for a male progenitor at all. The Director of the Womb Center's pitch is reminiscent of Firestone: 'No woman is completely free until she has control over her own reproductive system'.[94] Benefits for women are stated to include the freedom to find fulfilment in their careers without the burdens of pregnancy interfering, whereas for the foetus, it is repeatedly noted that they will be protected from stress, toxins, bacteria, etc. and experience 'optimized nutrition in a clean, safe, pure environment'.[95] For fathers, the pods are described as 'the closest thing a man is ever going to get' to experiencing gestation, as they are also able to 'carry' the pods around with them. When the film's protagonist, Rachel, asks a friend for advice on whether to contract the Womb Center's services, she and her partner, Alvy, are told:

> The uterus is a political issue … for decades women have not felt supported during their pregnancies … their pain minimized. Their symptoms dismissed as superficial! This has to stop. … It is the first time in history that, as women, we are not victims of our biology. Why would any of us want to feel nauseous and gain 35 pounds? Get stretch marks? … Progress has made all this unnecessary.[96]

The latter statement links with an earlier scene where employees asked whether the pervasive use of artificial intelligence (AI) in the workplace would mean their jobs were at risk, with their manager claiming: 'Progress has never made anyone redundant. It's here to help!'[97] However, in the case of reproduction, the technology depicted in *The Pod Generation* has arguably made many people redundant.

Although various statements are made in favour of more equal contributions to human reproduction, the 'nature knows best' theme is aggressively pursued throughout the film. Technology is shown to be disruptive and intrusive, Alvy describes a whole generation unable to 'interact with nature', claiming that the commodification of the natural world has left society 'emotionally starved', and Rachel describes the philosophy of the Womb Center as 'detachment parenting' and complains that she is unable to bond with her child.[98] While Alvy manages to connect with the 'pod baby' by taking it on a literal tree-hugging adventure, Rachel struggles to balance her work life with her impending motherhood, eventually running off to 'give birth' in the countryside, the lyrics of the background music repeating 'I'm beginning to see the light'.[99] Her dreams are full of 'natural pregnancy' images and beach scenes that are far removed from the artificial 'nature pod' sessions she attends at the direction of her AI therapist.

The Pod Generation also dramatizes some of the equity concerns regarding ectogenesis present in the literature, with several women of colour shown to be physically pregnant because they cannot afford access to the Womb Center. The company also blackmails parents and uses the developing foetuses to collect valuable research data, reminding parents that although the baby in the pod may be theirs, they do not own or control the patented technology in use. These latter interactions are perhaps the most ominous of the film, but the fixation on everything synthetic being a threat to human connection makes it clear that the feminist arguments being espoused are flawed and that deep down, women need to be physically pregnant to truly experience motherhood. Sexual equality may have been the achieved goal, but it has entailed significant loss for women, much like Piercy's characters describe the loss of gestation as a necessary sacrifice for the greater good of women's liberation.

As noted earlier, another famous example of this trope can be seen in Helen Sedgwick's *The Growing Season*, published in 2017 and set in an alternate reality version of 2016.[100] In this novel, prosthetic wombs are used to gestate offspring, with women, men and other kin able to share the responsibility of wearing the external 'pouch' device. The historical figure of Firestone is a revered celebrity in this alternate history, and sexual equality in reproduction is credited with the achievement of a more equitable distribution of social roles in society. However, just like in *The Pod Generation*, the company controlling the technology, FullLife, garners suspicion, and readers soon learn there are complications affecting the babies born from the pouch that are not being disclosed. Opponents of the pouch are also concerned with the societal effects of abandoning biological gestation, with the daughter of one of the leading anti-pouch activists recalling messages from her upbringing: 'We are women, her mother would say. Life grows inside of us, and we protect it'.[101] So even when the potential benefits of ectogenesis for equality are explicitly mentioned in science fiction, these are often counterbalanced by certain developmental issues for offspring and broader harms to society that rely on essentialist views of human reproduction.

Patterns of use of ectogenesis in science fiction

This final section aims to summarize the overall patterns of use of ectogenesis in science fiction and how this technology functions within the genre. As can be seen from the above examples, ectogenesis is often depicted negatively, both descriptively and visually, and even supposedly positive examples can be quite ambiguous. For example, using ectogenesis to create or maintain an army is unlikely to be met with universal support, even when painted in a positive light. While these descriptions and images can be tied to bioethical issues, as has been done above, it is important to consider how they function in science fiction as a genre. As has been noted, ectogenesis is rarely the central *novum*, in Suvinian terms, and in many cases is not essential to the science fiction plot. This, therefore, begs the question: why is it being incorporated at all? Lee M. Silver notes that in blueprint-style dystopias, like *Brave New World*, the purpose seems to be exploring how a reproductive technology could be co-opted by a state authority to the detriment of society and personal liberty.[102] He claims this is despite the fact '[i]t is individuals and couples … *not governments* – who will seize control of these new technologies' as these elements of society create 'the driving force behind babymaking'.[103] The science-fictional 'what if' here could be phrased: what if procreation fell entirely under the purview of the state instead of private individuals and couples? *Brave New World* plays out this fiction, demonstrating how such a future could lead to dystopia. By providing a map of what *not* to do, *Brave New World* implicates ectogenesis in its dystopian vision.

From within the science fiction genre, even when it is not essential to the plot, ectogenesis can be seen to contribute to the audience's estrangement, reminding them that what they are experiencing is distanced from the real world. As such, it forms part of the science fictionality of the science fiction text, even if it is rarely the defining characteristic making the text a work of science fiction, according to the criteria defended in the previous chapter. Aline Ferreira lists some additional purposes for ectogenesis within science fiction, noting:

> While ectogenesis stands at the root of a fantasy which could be equated with masculine womb envy, the dream of becoming a male mother and thus dispensing almost totally with women, for women, on the other hand, extra-uterine pregnancy, combined with cloning techniques, could constitute an enabling vision of autonomy from the male, but also a potentially threatening one.[104]

The various 'what ifs' represented in the above quote play out in single-gender fictional societies, such as in Bujold's *Ethan of Athos* (1986). These and other similar estranging effects of ectogenesis in science fiction will be considered in more detail in the final chapter.

4

Bioethics engaging with science fiction

This chapter will consider how science fiction has been used in discussions of emerging biotechnologies, including ectogenesis.[1] This will incorporate an exploration of the ways in which bioethicists and science communicators have used science fiction narratives, images and tropes in their writing and the potential impact of these stylistic choices on audiences. Tranter defines science fiction as 'the dreaming site for the West's technological futures, a place for working through both the anxieties and promises of technological change'.[2] Since the genre serves as a site to explore the scientific imaginary, the socio-political motivations behind its use in debates regarding emerging science and technologies warrant critical examination. As will be demonstrated in this chapter, although there is great potential for science fiction to promote balanced discussion of the ramifications of technological development on society, at present, its use predominantly favours a socially conservative political agenda.

The intersection between science fiction, bioethics and biopolitics

The study of bioethics relies heavily on the language and imagery of science fiction literature and film – particularly those texts from the utopian sub-genre – to debate such issues as what makes life meaningful, where the boundaries between the human and posthuman should be drawn and the ethical concerns surrounding certain medical and technological advances, including those that might impact these core elements of the human experience. As such, it is important to consider what this genre achieves for the rapidly expanding field of bioethics, both in terms of the potential for providing accessible philosophical arguments for public debate and the risks of fuelling sensationalist or negatively prejudiced images of emerging technologies. This chapter explores the use of science fiction in debates surrounding cloning, ectogenesis, genetic engineering and genetic discrimination, particularly focusing on three of the most commonly cited works of fiction in bioethics: Huxley's *Brave New World* (1932), Shelley's *Frankenstein; or, The Modern Prometheus* (1818) and Andrew Niccol's highly influential film, *Gattaca* (1997). These topics and texts were chosen due to the frequency of their use and the fact that they all intersect with the ectogenesis debate at different points. Existing both as philosophical thought experiments and socially conservative, technophobic cautionary tales, these texts serve a distinct political agenda when invoked in bioethics literature. Vint claims that biopolitics and science fiction speculation converge at the point at which political governance extends into biological life, with the intent of steering the future of that life.[3] Huxley's, Shelley's and Niccol's texts all represent leading examples of such a convergence in science fiction, relying on genre tropes to dramatize the potential threats science and technology may pose to humanity's freedom. The hubristic scientist 'playing God', science run amok, the inadvertent creation of monsters and life under bio-psycho-social totalitarianism are all effective propaganda against certain areas of scientific discovery, particularly reproductive biotechnology. These three texts also explore fictional worlds in which reproductive biotechnologies have fundamentally altered perceptions of human biology and reproduction. In *Brave New World*, widespread use of cloning and ectogenesis has almost completely replaced biological gestation (the exceptions being the naturally born 'savages' in the reservations).[4] Likewise, in *Gattaca*, every member of the fictional society must either engage in genetic engineering or have their offspring suffer the consequences of their failure to do so, including genetic discrimination in the workplace.[5] Shelley's classic horror *Frankenstein* functions as a proto-dystopia, a small-scale disruption to the familiar world, but one possessing the potential to have global consequences. Although the immediate horror of Frankenstein's monster is contained within his creator's personal interactions with him in the novel, the real cause for alarm is the potential for the monster to change the 'natural' balance of power in the world beyond this narrow sphere. In the end, Dr Victor Frankenstein does not actually create a 'race of devils' as he feared; however, the possibility of such a future race arising and challenging the supremacy of the human species remains a constant preoccupation throughout the novel.[6] When these texts appear in bioethics scholarship, it is always to advance a particular socio-political agenda. More often than not, such agendas are distinctly anti-technological.

With regard to their biopolitical significance, the above texts are not only concerned with who should have power over other people in general but also more specifically who should have the authority to direct the future of human biology. In *Frankenstein*, an individual scientist has usurped both God and Mother Nature; in *Brave New World*, the whole of human biology has fallen under the strict regulation of the state; and in *Gattaca*, the rule of the majority has institutionalized genetic discrimination through the normalization of population-wide genetic engineering programs. Each text also demonstrates the struggle for power over life and death that Michel Foucault identifies in *The History of Sexuality*. This power is imposed through regulatory control over the 'species body' and its reproductive functions, or what Foucault terms the *biopolitics of the population*.[7] Dr Frankenstein refuses to provide his monster a mate; the genetically enhanced in *Gattaca* have a competitive advantage in romantic pursuits; and the citizens in Huxley's World State have had all reproductive powers removed from them, with pharmaceutically induced pregnancy simulations being the closest any of them will experience to biological gestation. Power is also exerted through maximizing the efficiency or docility of the human body itself, demonstrating what Foucault terms the *anatomo-politics of the human body*.[8] In *Frankenstein*, the human physique is modified for strength; in *Gattaca*, the human genome is modified for health and in *Brave New World*, both the human body and psyche are modified for passive contentedness.[9] By depicting dystopian realities in this way, the targeted manipulation of the human form becomes the locus of a conservative resistance against the technoscience that made such manipulation possible. Thus, the use of these texts in bioethical debate is not only politically motivated but also forms part of the biopolitical discourse surrounding the integration of technology into existing and possible future socio-political power structures.

To explore the impact of these tactics further first requires a discussion of who is invoking science-fictional references when discussing new technologies. The next few sections consider how different stakeholders may engage with speculative fictions when discussing emerging reproductive biotechnologies, before narrowing the focus to the use by bioethicists specifically.

Science communicators and journalists using science fiction

It is perhaps not surprising that journalists and online bloggers wishing to sensationalize their articles on scientific advancements often invoke images of Frankensteinian monsters and dystopian futures, exploiting the anxieties of the general public for popularity and shock value. While such developments can be reported on in a neutral fashion, it is typical to engage some form of 'valence framing' intended to paint the relevant issue in a positive or negative light or provide some evaluative judgment on its associated socio-political ramifications.[10] Such framing has been shown to impact the strength of media consumers' attitudes of support or opposition to the issue being reported on and is often used as a tactic in election campaigns to rally support for a preferred candidate or consolidate feelings of negativity towards an opponent.[11] The technique can be found in both mainstream media and social media postings focused on reproductive biotechnologies, as seen in the examples below.

In September 1996, scientists in Tokyo announced they had successfully incubated a goat foetus in an artificial womb for up to three weeks. *The New York Times* gave the article the title 'The Artificial Womb is Born' and opened the piece with a quote from Huxley's *Brave New World*.[12] Without differentiating between animal and human foetuses, the chosen quote also included a reference to the 'Social Predestination Room', the site of government control over the population of Huxley's World State. Bearing no relevance to an artificially gestated goat foetus, it can only be assumed that the reference was intended to be associated with later comments in this news article predicting the generalizability of the described extrauterine foetal incubation (EUFI) technique to humans. *ConsciousNewsMedia* re-published this story in July 2013 from the *New York Times* archives, retaining the Huxley quote and extending the title to read: 'The Artificial Womb is Born and the World of the Matrix Begins', thus super-imposing the horrors of wide-scale human enslavement, destructive artificial intelligences and ecological apocalypse onto the image of the goat foetus growing in a tank.[13] As there is no inherent connection between EUFI and social oppression by either a totalitarian government or a race of sentient machines, these examples demonstrate both sensationalism and politically motivated valence framing, intent on strengthening oppositional attitudes and persuading consumers to abandon even tacit support of EUFI and other ectogenesis technologies.

A more recent example can be seen in the coverage of so-called 'synthetic embryos' in June 2023, with various news outlets reporting on the development with references to science fiction texts,[14] as they had done in 2021 when precursor animal models had been announced.[15] Ball's article for *The Guardian* noted some editorials also explicitly raised concerns about scientists 'playing god' or 'paving the way towards a dystopian 'Brave New World'''.[16] He labels the use of the misnomer 'synthetic embryo' as 'rather misleading, even prejudicial', again exposing the importance of language when dealing with novel entities, noting scientists preferred the more accurate term 'embryo models'.[17] It is hoped these models – created using stem cells instead of ova and sperm – may help unlock the 'black box' of early embryogenesis.[18] However, there is also the potential that they could be used in early ectogenesis trials to avoid the need for foetal experimentation. An interesting trend when comparing the news coverage of these embryo models to the previous example of goat foetuses undergoing artificial gestation is that some journalists quoted science fiction texts while simultaneously imploring their readers to avoid associating the relevant breakthroughs with these same texts. This contradiction is also seen in some legal scholarship focused on emerging technologies.

Lawyers and policymakers using science fiction

Tranter notes in his article 'The Speculative Jurisdiction: The Science Fictionality of Law and Technology' that lawyers and policymakers are also relying on science fiction references to debate the legal and bioethical issues surrounding possible future technologies. Paying particular attention to the issue of IVF, Tranter argues that lawyers in the 1970s and 1980s often treated this technology as a threatening 'next step' down the artificial human reproduction continuum, a progression they believed 'would end with cloning and ectogenesis'.[19] Since the creation of the world's first 'test-tube' baby, Louise Brown, had been prefigured in science fiction, Tranter claims '[i]t was almost mandatory for publishing on IVF and law to reference directly Huxley's *Brave New World* (1932) and Orwell's *Nineteen Eighty-Four* (1949)'.[20] It is noteworthy that both these texts are well known and distinctly dystopian. Tranter claims that such 'selective referencing' from within the genre has the potential to prejudice lawyers, policymakers and the public against certain biotechnologies by failing to appreciate the complexity of the issues being discussed.[21] Again, the association between Louise Brown's birth in 1978 and the rise of either of these dystopian futures is neither obvious nor justified; however, the use of Huxleyan and Orwellian imagery can be a persuasive tool influencing legal opinion towards reproductive biotechnologies.

When considering the ramifications of ectogenesis technologies on the legality of abortion in 1979 for the *Arizona Law Review*, Robert J. Favole identified a lack of detailed scientific writing on the topic to assist lawyers and policymakers in decision-making. Referencing Laurence E. Karp's book *Genetic Engineering: Threat or Promise?*, Favole claimed that this lack of available research was the result of 'hostile attitudes' towards ectogenesis in the general public brought on by repeated association with Huxley's *Brave New World*.[22] In addition to such specific textual references in legal scholarship, there are also general references to science fiction as a genre that do not single out individual texts. For example, in her discussion of the legal status of cryopreserved embryos for the *Cardoza Journal of Law and Gender*, Bridget M. Fuselier outlines a scenario in which a daughter inherits her mother's frozen embryos and intends to gestate her genetic siblings against their father's wishes. Noting the lack of legal direction currently available for such a case, Fuselier claims such a 'science-fiction soap opera' demonstrates the need to establish policies regarding legal rights over unimplanted embryos.[23] Similarly, as noted in Chapter 3, writing for the *Southern California Law Review* Cohen labels his 'bathtub case', in which a person is unknowingly made a genetic parent after their skin cells have been harvested from a hotel bathtub, as a 'science fiction thought experiment' designed to illustrate the need to clearly delineate the level of voluntariness required in a procreative project for the law to impose legal parenthood on a genetic parent.[24] In both of these instances, the authors go on to warn readers that such speculative fictions are fast becoming possible realities, but the process by which their dystopian predictions may come true remains vague and unconvincing. The invocation of science fiction as some nebulous entity also accounts for much of its use in scientific literature, as will be explored next.

Scientists and researchers using science fiction

One of the most interesting discoveries when exploring who is using science fiction to describe new reproductive biotechnologies is the extent to which scientists themselves use these references when communicating their research. While many accuse journalists of distorting the scientific facts in their comparisons between emerging technologies and popular science fiction imagery, Hamilton notes that following the successful cloning of Dolly the sheep in 1996, both her creator, Dr Ian Wilmut, and leading bioethicist and biologist, Lee M. Silver, released statements containing references to science fiction. With Wilmut defending his position that 'cloning people should be in the realm of science fiction' and Silver declaring that now 'all of science fiction is true',[25] what Hamilton finds most revealing about these examples, like several of the law examples provided above, is the lack of specificity regarding the genre:

> Why, however, would both these figures so prominently invoke science fiction? In making their claims, these scientists are doing something that at first glance

> might seem unlikely: they are directly linking biotechnological science with science fiction. Significantly, neither is referencing a particular sf novel, film or television program; both evoke the genre as a broader cultural trope. This rhetorical tactic seems curious in that science fiction might not necessarily be the best way to promote the credibility of science, particularly biotechnology, which commentators have noted has serious public relations problems.[26]

In his statement against human cloning, Wilmut is reaffirming that certain scientific ideas rightly belong *solely* in the fictional utopias of the scientific imaginary. Meanwhile, Silver is using the public's familiarity with science fiction tropes to suggest that the advent of a cloned sheep demonstrates that the boundary between fact and fiction has collapsed – in short, if a human mind can conceive of a given technology, science can now make it a reality. While this is clearly an overstatement, whether a reader is likely to fear or take comfort from such a pronouncement will depend on the types of science fiction stories they have been exposed to, with the most thoroughly culturally engrained examples often tending towards dystopia and horror.

At the time these statements were released, exposure to at least one science fiction narrative was practically a given. When discussing Dolly, *Brave New World* references abounded in popular and news media, legal and bioethics scholarship and even scientific literature, with both Dr Frankenstein and his monster also making numerous appearances. According to Jane Maienschein, what became 'very clear very quickly' following the entrance of Dolly into the cloning debate 'was the importance of words and perspective'.[27] She claims the initial response of the US Congress to the possibilities that Dolly represented was a 'frightened reaction to the idea of runaway Frankenstein-like scientists copying people in their labs'.[28] Given this fear, it is again surprising that scientists would invite such reflections by referencing science fiction themselves.

In their article, 'An Empirical Revision of the Definition of Science Fiction', Christopher Benjamin Menadue et al. claim that:

> Researchers employ science fiction and fantasy in public engagement, advocacy, and education as significant sources of insights to identify public interests, inspire public policy, and influence future science. These uses of science fiction as a source that is expected to reflect public interests are undermined if the examples employed by researchers are interpreted differently by the intended audience or beneficiaries of research.[29]

These authors refer to Jesse Weiner et al.'s 2018 description of science fiction as 'a crucial and popular mode, even *the* mainstream mode, of thinking about life in a modern technoscientific world'[30] to explain why researchers are often motivated to use science-fictional references when communicating their work.[31] Some examples can be seen in University of Melbourne scientists discussing the imaginative possibilities of science fiction leading to real-world innovation in an interview for their university newsletter in 2017, with physicist, Steven Prawar, linking research into bionic vision to *Star Trek: The Next Generation*'s chief engineer, Lieutenant Commander Georgi La Forge, who wears a high-tech 'visor' due to congenital blindness.[32] Meanwhile biohacking researcher, Kayla Heffernan, claims many members of the public fear implantable microchips due to misconceptions gleaned from *Total Recall* about the government using such devices to track the population, with reporter Kate Stanton instead suggesting that opening a door with an implanted microchip is more like the telekinesis displayed by *Stranger Things* character, Eleven. Human-robot relations researcher, Denny Oetomo, then bemoans how difficult the public are to impress, given their familiarity with robots from *iRobot* and *Star Wars* which have for years displayed capabilities that have only recently become a reality in robotics laboratories, with biomedical engineer, David Grayden, similarly noting that *The Six Million Dollar Man* and *Bionic Woman* have exaggerated the possible functionality of real-world bionic implants.[33] Throughout these accounts, these researchers indicate an enchantment with science fiction that inspires scientists to continue pushing the boundaries of what is possible, even when simultaneously expressing concern that the public's knowledge may be unduly influenced by unrealistic fictional science. These concerns about scientific accuracy also feature in some bioethicists' engagement with peers who draw on science fiction in bioethical debate.

Bioethicists using science fiction

While certainly not a practice adopted by all bioethicists, many will use science fiction language and motifs to frame their arguments, especially regarding novel technologies. Some notable examples include Leon Kass, Ronald M. Green and Nicholas Agar – with the latter's seminal work, *Liberal Eugenics*, containing one reference to *Frankenstein*, nine to *Gattaca* and the phrase 'Brave New World' at least three times.[34] Similarly, when writing on scientism versus Luddism for *American Journal of Bioethics*, Nancy C. Jones equates Luddism with the fear that scientific advancements will lead to 'a reincarnated Frankenstein, deviously plotting to take over the world and create Aldous Huxley's *Brave New World*'.[35]

This quotation demonstrates the practice Hamilton observed of drawing on science fiction as a 'broader cultural trope', with the relevance of the two unrelated narratives being neither explicitly stated nor concerned with any degree of textual fidelity. Thus, it is not just science fiction tropes but also science fiction *as a trope* that have become important touchstones in bioethics scholarship. The invocation of the genre tends to be dismissive and/or derogatory, while the use of individual texts often oscillates between vague negativity or specific threat. All three common uses fail to capitalize on science fiction's potential to fill an important role in mediating between different stakeholders in humanity's reproductive future.

Focusing on bioethicists' use of *Brave New World* first, Chris Mason notes this cautionary tale is often referenced as a means of exploring the potential social impact of emerging reproductive biotechnologies on traditional views of sex, reproduction and family.[36] Many writers using *Brave New World* do not directly quote from the text though, but rather rely on generalized conceptions of the text and its meaning. Used as an argument against both cloning and ectogenesis, a closer textual analysis of *Brave New World* reveals that the core of the dystopia is one of government-mandated social stratification and conditioning that owes very little to either of these technologies. A good example can be seen in Ted Peters and Gaymon Bennet Jr.'s review of the ethical implications of cloning and stem cell research, in which they identify three competing bioethical frameworks used to discuss these issues, one of which is simply labelled the 'anti-Brave New World'.[37] They claim that by invoking dystopian images of a Huxleyan future, proponents of this technologically conservative philosophy can successfully prejudice the public against a variety of biotechnological developments, many of which could yield significant health benefits for the population.

A similar approach is taken by Kass, whose extensive use of science fiction references to argue matters of ethical importance has led to some criticism from rival philosophers. S. Philip Morgan et al. claim that Kass's use of *Brave New World* as representative of the inevitable future of a society that permits human cloning, while certainly managing to frighten his readers, bears little resemblance to Huxley's actual text.[38] What is of interest here is not the level of textual fidelity, or lack thereof, found in these arguments, but rather their common assumption that all of their readers will at least be vaguely familiar with the dystopian future Huxley imagined. That the language and imagery of *Brave New World* has infiltrated the bioethical literature on cloning to such an extent that an entire ethical framework can be reduced to 'anti-Brave New World' is evidence that utopian fiction and bioethics have become firmly entwined.

While praised for being accessible to a wide audience, Green's reliance on utopian science fiction in his argument against allowing 'babies by design'[39] is also criticized for an over-dependence on negative portrayals of cloning and genetic engineering in science-fictional texts, such as *Brave New World* and *Gattaca*. Dena S. Davis claims that by using these dystopian projections of the future as a frame of reference for discussing current and advancing medical technologies, Green allows popular culture to paint these developments in a negative light, rather than providing persuasive ethical arguments to oppose them.[40] It is important to remember that most of the science fiction texts appearing in bioethics literature depict technological change negatively, with positive counter-examples often lacking. Hilary S. Crew openly questions how different social attitudes towards cloning might be, were there another text as widely known as *Brave New World* that speculated on the potential benefits such technology could bring society.[41]

When it comes to ectogenesis, association with this dystopian text conflates the issues surrounding artificial gestation with those of human cloning and the bio-psycho-social totalitarianism of Huxley's World State, with its prenatally conditioned, drug-addled population and the total abolition of the traditional family unit. What can be observed now is a kind of feedback loop, in which *Brave New World*'s popularity was originally owed to the fact that it spoke to contemporary concerns regarding the future of human reproduction but now, in turn, provides the very foundation of that concern in the present. Even if an author or reader does not truly know the alternative reality depicted in *Brave New World*, they know that it is *bad*. Thus, while science fiction has the potential to engender a sense of scientific and technological enchantment, such selective use of *Brave New World* in bioethics literature can be seen as perpetuating a certain scepticism and disenchantment towards science and particularly reproductive biotechnology.[42] As Tranter notes, 'dystopian science fiction can be seen as profoundly anti-technological', and dystopias account for the majority of the science fiction texts being used in both legal and bioethical debate, especially regarding ectogenesis.[43]

While relying on the cultural cache of Huxley's classic dystopia to substitute for considered debate may be scholastically lazy, Jenny Kitzinger argues it is similarly problematic to simply dismiss public concern about emerging biotechnologies because citizens may have been influenced by speculative fictions.[44] In her article, 'Questioning the Sci-Fi Alibi', she claims that despite many people referencing *Brave New World* and *Frankenstein* when discussing novel technologies, there is not a 'simple causal relationship' between public understanding of science and negative depictions in fiction.[45] For this study, she said she used 'the term "science fiction" not in the academic form – to refer to a specific genre – but as a short hand embracing a range of fictional representations of science. This short hand reflects the way in which scientists and policy-makers criticising fiction often use the term'.[46] While the participants in her empirical audience research were mostly able to differentiate truth from fiction, Kitzinger did find a minority of respondents had 'clearly been misled by science fiction representations'.[47] She notes science fiction references are often metaphorical, dismissive or used to construct a 'straw man', however, even here, it is admitted that certain areas of science are more likely to be negatively impacted by misuse of fiction than others, with stem cell research and cloning being particularly vulnerable.[48] As such, the use of science-fictional references when discussing these topics in bioethics may require additional attention and careful consideration.

Moving on to the use of *Frankenstein* in bioethics scholarship, this text appears most frequently in discussions of genetic engineering, including for plants, animals and humans, and in articles focused on novel reproductive biotechnologies.[49] Regarding the former, Anne Murcott bemoans the repeated use of the term 'Frankenfoods' to describe genetically modified crops, claiming that public opinion has been manipulated so artfully through its usage that 'science fiction and science fact' can no longer be distinguished.[50] This is a view shared by many other stakeholders in the industry, with bioengineers protesting against accusations of hubris and irresponsibleness, with the image of the scientist 'playing God' being a common trope borrowed from science fiction. The catastrophic predictions for genetically engineered plants and animals are often attributed to fictional sources, where the acceptance of such technologies at this early stage often represents a 'slippery slope', which inevitably leads to genetic enhancements for humans (Franken-babies!),[51] the development of a genetic underclass (as in the society depicted in *Gattaca*),[52] or to ecological apocalypse (killer corn!).[53] However, Emma Hughes and Jenny Kitzinger claim that while policymakers express concern about 'such pervasive references to fiction and their impact on public discussion about emerging science and technologies such as GM crops', that hard evidence for fiction's supposed 'corrosive influence on science literacy' is often lacking.[54] These authors admit that science fiction's treatment of emerging technologies is often considered 'technophobic' or even 'regressive', and that science-fictional images 'can *sometimes* be a primary source of an image of a technology'; nevertheless, they claim science fiction references are often used by the public 'with distance, humour, and irony', suggesting a more nuanced relationship than some commentators assume.[55] For something microscopic and hard to otherwise imagine, like experiments within the field of genetics, the absence of other recognizable images might make something that looms as large as Frankenstein's monster a more plausibly persuasive image source. For a technology that only currently exists within science fiction, like ectogenesis, the same rule may apply.

According to G. Pascal Zachary, the persistent image of scientific creations developing a 'mind of their own' and bringing about the downfall of their creators 'owes a lot to the image of Frankenstein's monster'.[56] For obvious reasons, Shelley's original text contains no reference to genetic engineering, cloning or stem cell research, but these are the bioethical and biopolitical debates in which Dr Frankenstein and his creature are most frequently found today. Leaving aside the common misappropriation of the name of Shelley's protagonist to represent a scientifically manipulated product (which in the text is the unnamed monster), the presence of references to *Frankenstein* in these debates speaks to the adaptability of Shelley's work and the timelessness of societal concerns regarding the risks of 'playing God' and defying nature through boundary-free science. More specifically, the text can be seen to warn against handing over the power to direct humanity's biological future to a subset of humans, whether scientists or state officials.

Associating any future reproductive biotechnology with the stereotypical 'mad scientist', Dr Frankenstein, automatically infers a moral judgment against that technology and those who would seek to develop and control it. There is also a clear message contained in such references; as Mason notes, Dr. Frankenstein's 'transgressions into anthropoeia' cost him greatly, and the moral of the story is clearly focused on respecting – rather than pushing – the boundaries of nature and science.[57] Given the cultural impact of Shelley's work, the term 'Frankensteinian' when applied to any branch of science must necessarily carry with it strong connotations of moral disapprobation. Thus, when describing scientific breakthroughs and including references to *Frankenstein*, bioethicists are not critically engaging with Shelley's novel but rather capitalizing on its cultural currency to support a particular socio-political argument, usually one opposed to a given area of scientific research. Mason's argument also references various other texts described in Chapter 3, including *Splice*, *The Matrix* and *The Island*, noting the influence of these films on public perceptions of scientific research.[58]

In their article, 'Dr Frankenstein's Bioethical Experiment', for *The Lancet*, Ann Jurecic and Daniel Marchalik note:

> Shelley's story has been used many times since its publication to express fears about new technologies and the risks of scientific overreach – fears that were later often recognised as unfounded. Frankenstein was evoked with regard to organ transplantation in the mid-20th century, in-vitro fertilisation in the 1970s, and genetically engineered 'Frankenfoods' and animal cloning in the 1990s. Today, the gene editing technology CRISPR has aroused concerns in some quarters about the effects of tampering with human genomes.[59]

Regarding the latter point, claims that the Chinese scientist, He Jiankui, had used CRISPR-Cas9 to edit the genome of babies Lulu and Nana to make them resistant to HIV infection shocked the world in 2018. News outlets labelled him 'China's gene-editing "Frankenstein"', while bioethicists scrambled to respond to this new reality.[60] Derek So's 2022 article for *Bioethics* notes that although germline editing has been a topic of conversation in science and ethics for some time, due to the lack of any genetically modified humans until very recently, public expectations of the traits such people would express relied on accounts from 'genetics research, associations with other reproductive technologies, or even science fiction tropes'.[61] He claims that since 'schemas are based on experience', and no experience of CRISPR-modified humans was previously available, these sources provided alternatives to aid comprehension.[62] Adam J. Gross's earlier comment for *Jurimetrics*, entitled 'Dr. Frankenstein, Or: How I Learned to Stop Worrying and Love CRISPR-Cas9', approaches the same issue from the angle of international regulation (outlining various legal options from international conventions), self-regulation (comparing this to the goal of the Asilomar conference focused on recombinant DNA in the 1970s), to the use of certain United Nations instruments to promote human dignity.[63] Ultimately, he concludes that international regulatory systems will fail and citizens will have 'little choice but to trust CRISPR-Cas9 users and to know that the catastrophic, doomsday scenarios that occur in the imaginations of science fiction authors are so unlikely that they are nearly impossible'.[64] Nevertheless, the spectre of Frankenstein's monster has attached itself to discussions of CRISPR technologies, with various bioethicists seemingly encouraging this association in their writing.[65]

Finally, considering the film, *Gattaca*, David A. Kirby claims this film is 'an example of an extrapolative science fiction' in which the 'filmmakers act as bioethicists'.[66] He notes the strong influence science fiction can have on public perceptions of scientific development, explaining why *Gattaca* features so prominently in debates about the ethics of genetic susceptibility testing in the workplace, the risks of genetic discrimination and the flaws inherent in genetic determinism. Kirby claims that science fiction 'provides scholars a gauge of social concerns, social attitudes, and social change regarding science and technology'.[67] Lee Easton further argues that, as such speculative fictions are 'neither simply social commentary nor precise scientific prediction', films like *Gattaca* can become part of the discourse determining our cultural response to new technologies.[68] By dramatizing ethical dilemmas rather than lecturing about them, science fiction can both educate and entertain, drawing on abstracted philosophical arguments to achieve real-world socio-political goals.

In 'Lifting the Genetic Veil of Ignorance: Is There Anything Really Unjust about Gattacan Society?', Sandra Shapshay uses *Gattaca* to illustrate the potential threat posed by unregulated genetic technologies on equality of opportunity in a near-future American society. Opposing those critics who claim the warnings about genetic discrimination in *Gattaca* are 'overblown', Shapshay continues by discussing what she finds the most insidious aspect of *Gattaca*: the unintentional creation of a eugenicist society through the release of genetic enhancement technologies as personal services that couples 'can take or leave' as they desire.[69] When invoked in bioethics literature, the name *Gattaca* alone can serve as a warning against the dangers of developing a society that is dependent on what Curtis A. Kin labels a legalized 'genetic supermarket'.[70] Unlike in *Brave New World*, *Gattaca* does not rely on state interference and control over human reproduction to produce a dystopia; in fact, the non-interference of the state can be seen as part of the problem, as it tolerates the perpetuation of unequal employment opportunities for those citizens existing outside the genetically enhanced bourgeoisie.

When considering the relevance of this film to the ectogenesis debate, Lantos and Janvier recall that Haldane's original vision for artificial gestation included pursuing a eugenicist agenda:

> He imagined that we would harvest eggs and sperm from the small proportion of men and women who were superior in musical taste and intelligence in order to amplify the proportion of their genes in the population. While eugenics has been disgraced, many eugenic ideas have resurfaced as justifications for prenatal diagnosis, in vitro fertilization, and pre-implantation genetic diagnosis.[71]

The stain of this legacy goes some way towards explaining the common association between ectogenesis and genetic engineering, despite the fact that the latter technology focuses on conception, rather than gestation.

In Niccol's film, the ethical implications of allowing directed human evolution and eugenics to be practised freely in society are well described, with *Gattaca* potentially representing one of the only frames of reference many people have for considering the social and political implications of genetic technology. By encouraging sympathy for the unenhanced 'in-Valids' of the Gattacan society, viewers can become politicized on the issue of genetic discrimination, a topic they may not have previously had any interest in or knowledge about. In this case, resistance is not framed as rebellion against a powerful government, but rather as a duty to oppose the development of a technology that, if made available to individuals and couples, would serve to perpetuate social inequality. According to Silver, this makes the film a more realistic vision of the future than Huxley's dystopia, as it recognizes that prospective parents are the ones who will use some reproductive technologies 'to reach otherwise unattainable reproductive goals and others to help their children achieve health, happiness, and success'.[72] Thus, the problems in *Gattaca* are facilitated by liberal legislation but promoted by a free market economy.

Having considered the various groups who may use science-fictional references when discussing emerging technologies, the next few sections will cover various motivations behind these references.

Science fiction as warning

There are many reasons why science fiction lends itself to discussions on the nature of science and technology, and various motives for employing the language and imagery of the genre in bioethical and biopolitical debates. As the examples above demonstrate, whether someone has personally read *Brave New World*, *Frankenstein*, or watched *Gattaca*, there is an assumption when using these texts in debate that most members of the public will have a basic knowledge of the central issues arising in these texts. These include warnings against trusting the hubristic and fallible scientist or the seemingly benevolent state authorities, the threat of unleashing the monstrously ugly and the potential horrors of interfering with nature. Taking the example of *Frankenstein*, over two centuries since its creation, Shelley's horror classic still has resonance when applied to bioethical discussion, associating certain research projects with the potential for grotesque and usually unforeseen side effects. Wolpert claims that Shelley would be both 'proud and shocked' at the impact her novel continues to have, both as a means of approaching concerns regarding scientific progress and for its ability to condemn entire research proposals through the mere mention of its name.[73] Here, it is the popular conceptualization of *Frankenstein*, and not any in-depth analysis of the text, that is substituting for informed philosophical debate. In this way, the characters in *Frankenstein* transcend their original text, and association with them can automatically force one side of a bioethical debate onto the defensive.

In her 2009 editorial, 'More Than Cautionary Tales: The Role of Fiction in Bioethics', Sarah Chan notes:

> Science fiction may sometimes be used to articulate fears over science without really exploring or drawing attention to the deeper ethical questions … but nevertheless creators of fiction should be wary of resorting to scaremongering and sensationalism in their pursuit of a good story. … Fiction, then, can be unethical in the sense of being against ethics when it reinforces irrational fears or false beliefs. Such misdirection may have serious negative consequences if it turns the public against science that would otherwise produce benefits in terms of human wellbeing.[74]

Such an argument may be particularly compelling in the case of ectogenesis and other emerging reproductive biotechnologies that have the potential to promote alternative methods of family creation. In these instances, using science fiction as a warning may be contributing to the poverty of imagination currently restricting the development of these technologies, including those that could substantially benefit women and members of the LGBTIQ+ community. Contrasting Chan's claims, some may argue it is not the fiction author's job to ensure realistic or fair depictions of scientific development; however, the same cannot be said for science communicators or bioethicists. Among these professionals, exploiting public fears in a way that hinders scientific development cannot be excused on the grounds of entertainment. Using *Brave New World* as an example, Chan claims that within bioethics scholarship, this text is 'seemingly cited in perpetuity whenever the cloning debate arises', further noting:

> The subject matter of bioethical discussions often borders on the territory of speculative or science fiction. Human cloning, animal-human hybrids and genetic engineering have all found a place in fictional as well as bioethical literature. Similarly, creatures and concepts from science fiction populate bioethical debate, albeit sometimes as a form of metaphorical shorthand for an underlying argument.[75]

This is reminiscent of Chambers' argument regarding the narrative nature of bioethics outlined in Chapter 2, with Chan agreeing that fiction can replace traditional thought experiments and case studies.[76] The next section will further explore how this metaphorical shorthand can develop and be used in bioethical debate.

Science fiction providing a shared language of metaphors and names

As a speculative genre, science fiction can depict things that do not exist outside of the imagination. Hellsten claims that science fiction tropes can serve as metaphors for discussing science and technology, focusing the public's attention on specific areas of bioethical concern in a way that supports particular political agendas.[77] She notes that scientific discoveries are often framed in public debate as either 'sensational breakthroughs and innovations' or as 'steps toward creating new Frankensteins', claiming the latter argument deliberately uses this science fiction imagery to 'block some aspects of the issue out of focus'.[78] Some emerging reproductive biotechnologies, including ectogenesis, are currently subject to blanket bans in many countries, despite wide-ranging potential benefits. There is a need to establish a justification for banning scientific development in this area that speaks to common public concerns, but for this to occur, the public needs to be able to understand the ramifications of scientific advancement on society and the biopolitical implications of increased state and private interference in biological life. Maienschein notes that when engaging members of the public in discussions concerning policy regulation of scientific endeavours, a 'familiar and conventionally accepted language' must be available.[79] This is where science fiction can assist communication by providing a shared language to aid the dissemination of scientific knowledge and political opinion. As Vint argues: 'understanding the speculative discourses of biopolitics is imperative, and sf is in a privileged position to help us think through its anxieties and contradictions'.[80] However, without balanced representation, such understanding will remain elusive.

As addressed earlier, bioethics represents a point of intersection between science and the humanities, scientists and the public. It is interesting that popular culture references have become part of the common language for such encounters, especially considering that the language of philosophy at large is not generally deemed to be particularly accessible. However, while some areas of philosophy deal in more abstract terms, the issues being decided upon in bioethical discussions can have real-world and immediate impact on all citizens, thus demonstrating the need to involve the general public in these discussions. Hamilton claims that science fiction provides an opportunity to reflect on science, and that the 'persistent presence' of references to the genre in literature discussing emerging biotechnologies is 'highly significant in terms of how cultural meanings of biotechnologies are constructed'.[81] Squier and Heather Latimer both go further to argue that fictional representations of reproductive biotechnologies are actually creating the social and cultural conditions for the posthuman.[82] Science fiction achieves this goal by abandoning the constraints of the physical world and exploring alternative realities in which the posthuman already exists. Thus, the power of fiction in bioethical debates stems from writers being able to make issues come alive through the creation of imaginary characters that appeal to audiences' sympathies – putting a name to the posthuman face, so to speak. It has been well documented that the specific name given to an entity has a significant impact on how that entity is treated,[83] which explains how referring to the cloned, genetically engineered or artificially gestated children of the future as 'Brave New Worlders'[84] or 'Franken-babies' can serve to manipulate public opinion regarding the associated reproductive biotechnologies. As outlined in Chapter 1, one of the prevailing issues in ectogenesis scholarship presently relates to establishing appropriate terminology.

Providing common ground for bioethical discussion through shared language and metaphors is valuable, but there is a concern when the metaphor *becomes* the argument or unduly biases the discussion. For example, Chan relates the results of a survey of the Dutch population in which ninety-one per cent said they opposed cloning, and sixty-four per cent 'cited as a reason for their opposition the 1978 movie *The Boys from Brazil*'.[85] That the clones in this film all turn out to be violent might be prejudicial enough; however, the fact they are specifically Hitler clones assures they are perceived negatively. As bioethicist Gregory E. Pence claims, 'many misconceptions about human cloning come from science fiction. At least half of this fiction sees human clones as little better than troglodytes … People who create humans by cloning in fiction have evil motives and their creations cause evil'.[86] This is certainly the case in *The Boys from Brazil* (1978), where both the clones and their creator are involved in a sinister plot to re-instate the Third Reich. This again highlights that it is not only the science from science fiction that appears in bioethics but also the socio-political thought experimentation Suvin considered inherent to the utopian sub-genre. The next section considers the potential pedagogical value of such discussion points.

Science fiction as bioethical and biopolitical instruction

Science fiction narratives can also serve as educational tools for teaching bioethics and biopolitics. For example, if asked to explain what genetic discrimination is, many among the uninitiated may struggle to come up with a definition, let alone an argument. However, when asked to elucidate the problem depicted in the Gattacan society, these same people can identify the elements of genetic discrimination as they affect Vincent, *Gattaca*'s unenhanced protagonist. For this reason, Silver advises all geneticists to watch *Gattaca*, 'if for no other reason than to understand the perception … of the public-at-large' toward genetic engineering.[87] This film also demonstrates that, although the use of enhancing technologies in the future may be voluntary, access will still most likely be restricted to those financially able to pay for them, dramatizing the ethical dilemma of allowing a society of genetic 'haves' and 'have nots' to develop. As noted in Chapter 2, science fiction can communicate the potential implications of technoscience through engaging audiences in moral spectatorship and imaginative work, including the equity and justice concerns associated with advanced medical technologies.

Françoise Baylis and Jason Scott Robert claim that genetic engineering will inevitably lead to genetic enhancements, 'because so many of us are crass capitalists, eager to embrace biocapitalism'.[88] These authors further argue that genetic enhancements 'will never be available on demand' and thus have the potential to shatter the 'myth of equality of opportunity' that many cultures rely on to secure social cooperation among citizens.[89] This is due to the fact that instead of promoting the idea that anyone can achieve success through hard work, genetic technologies will mean the socially privileged will be born with enhancements that place the unenhanced at even greater disadvantage in competition. *Gattaca* is thus seen by some as a call-to-arms for policymakers and the public to fight against this kind of future.[90] Furthermore, the film explores the question of genuine choice regarding accessing reproductive biotechnologies, by suggesting that once a technology is available, there will automatically be social pressure to use it. Take, for example, how IVF has influenced societal attitudes towards infertility (and in some places also adoption), and it becomes clear that scientific advancement has the potential to alter our perceptions of the biological 'norm'. As is currently the case for IVF, the socio-political motivations governing the provision of future reproductive biotechnology services, including genetic therapies, will also warrant close examination by all stakeholders. Extrapolating to full ectogenesis, the existence of this technology in the future may fundamentally alter how obstacles to gestation are viewed, for example, being born without a uterus or having had an emergency hysterectomy. Where surrogacy or adoption were previously the 'solution' to such barriers, ectogenesis could become the new norm, just as IVF has been normalized as the answer to tubal damage.

As another educational practice, science fiction is well suited to contribute to 'bioethics-in-literature' methodologies, where narratives are used to illustrate and explore ethical dilemmas and principles. When it comes to using this method in the bioethics classroom, Howard Brody notes bioethicists are often happy to teach ethical concepts using 'snappy short stories', but fewer engage with longer literary examples.[91] When considering using popular culture in bioethical instruction more broadly, Juan Jorge Michel Fariña relates this practice to Aristotelian and Platonic understandings of the power of rhetoric:

> Through cinematic resources, the idea and its argumentative development (logos) is strengthened by evoking passions and sentiments (pathos) using music, images, movement, and poetry through the framework of a process of genuine transmission from teacher to audience (ethos).[92]

This is again similar to Cartwright's moral spectatorship described in Chapter 2.[93] In their article, 'Medical Ethics through the Star Trek Lens', James J. Hughes and John D. Lantos focus attention solely on the science fiction genre, suggesting it is not through developing argumentation, but rather simply by relating ethical concepts in a dramatic format that imparts valuable knowledge, stating:

> Somehow, the fairy tale aspect of the science fiction allows difficult moral issues to be raised and analyzed without the intellectual paralysis that sometimes comes from trying to raise the same issues in the abstract. … we find the dramatization of ethical issues, rather than the philosophic explication of those same issues, to have pedagogic value.[94]

Both these possible uses of bioethics-in-literature methodology will be explored in the next chapter after a brief consideration of the role of science-fictional world-building on ethical communication.

Science fiction providing 'worlds of reference' to explore

The final use of science fiction in bioethics to be considered here relates to the genre's ability to promote discussion of ethical concerns in an ostensibly non-biased hypothetical environment. Hughes and Lantos note that by creating a fictional reality that distances audiences from the real world, moral and ethical dilemmas can be illustrated in a way that allows 'generalizability without insisting upon it'.[95] They compare this role to that which is performed by the 'philosophical parable', claiming science fiction is able to analyse the same issues as those addressed by the hypothetical 'mental exercises' of philosophical debate, but in less abstract terms.[96] For these authors, the significant impact science fiction has on public opinion earns the genre the label of socio-political thought experiments – artificial scenarios with real-world pedagogic value. Through the debates surrounding reproductive biotechnologies, there are often repeated reminders that the possibilities depicted in science fiction are fast becoming realities, and that the public needs to be aware of the potential risks of certain scientific advancements. The media frenzy often accompanying major developments in biotechnology demonstrates the role the genre can play in public education, as many science fiction texts have already thoroughly explored the possible socio-political ramifications of emerging technologies well before the creation of a successful prototype. Taking the example of *Brave New World*, it was before the widespread acceptance of IVF that Huxley's future prediction dominated the literature on this topic, as there were no real-world examples of human societies that used this technology that could be pointed to. Now there is evidence that IVF babies pose no immediate threat to democracy or human liberty, *Brave New World*'s use has mostly shifted to the cloning and ectogenesis debates, maintaining this element of *future* speculation. John D. Biggers notes that between the first successful attempt to culture pre-implantation mammalian embryos in 1913 and the first public lecture by Haldane on the possibility for *in vitro* reproductive technologies to lead to artificial gestation in 1923, discussions of this technology were almost entirely contained within the realm of utopian science fiction.[97] Furthermore, Biggers claims that the idea of ectogenesis only became 'widely disseminated' through the publication of *Brave New World* in 1932, thereby introducing this concept to the public.[98] Even today, the fictional worlds of science fiction still represent the only place human ectogenesis currently exists.

With regard to the cloning debate, Patrick D. Hopkins claims there is a 'Brave New Rhetoric' in bioethical literature that is dependent not on Huxley's actual book but on the 'trope connected with the book'.[99] Vague references to the dystopia depicted in *Brave New World* are even used to stand in for philosophical argument entirely by those attempting to expose the potential risks of allowing the state to exercise political governance over human reproductive biology through the application of science. As Firchow notes:

> So deep a mark has this work left on the modern literate mind that the mere mention of it evokes a whole complex of hostile attitudes towards science. It has become a kind of byword for a society in which the values (or nonvalues) of scientific technology are dominant, and which has therefore reduced man to a species of machines.[100]

It is difficult to imagine what the world might look like with the integration of the posthuman into human society. Cloning and ectogenesis, for example, carry with them a challenge to traditional views of parenthood and family, with Huxley's fictional society providing one possible scenario in which these challenges have essentially obliterated familial affection. Ethical concerns regarding reproductive biotechnologies often focus on the threat such techniques pose to the concept of the biological family unit, while also addressing the issue of the commodification of human life, and the predicted loss of individuality, autonomy and dignity this would entail. The inhabitants of Huxley's dystopia allow for the personification of these bioethical issues in the context of a totalitarian state. It also illustrates that although technology itself may be politically neutral, its application and regulation rarely are.[101] This lesson can be very effectively taught through exploring either *Brave New World*'s government control of human reproduction or *Gattaca*'s social policing of directed evolution. However, when hoping to explore the potential for ectogenesis and other emerging reproductive technologies to promote sexual equality in human reproduction, the world-building in *Woman on the Edge of Time* (1976) is more valuable, with Piercy's utopia, Mattapoisett, representing an alternative human society without the restrictive gender norms impacting women in the real world. Martin Thomasson thus suggests, 'Mattapoisett is Piercy's utopian vision of a community in which technology is used reflectively and caringly to enhance the lives of its inhabitants'.[102]

Lawyers and bioethicists both lament the fact that the legal and ethical implications of new reproductive biotechnologies are often not sufficiently explored before they are released, with some claiming they emerge in a moral and legal 'vacuum'.[103] Science fiction speculation can bridge this gap by exploring the socio-political issues facing possible future societies, particularly those encountering technologies with the potential to radically alter perceptions of the nature of humanity and definitions of human reproduction. Thus, the bioethical issues associated with new scientific discoveries can provide narrative fodder for fiction authors, while the characters these authors create can provide analogies for bioethicists for future people living in a world in which currently emerging biotechnologies are fully realized. As will be discussed in the next chapter, the narrative point of view adopted for these stories will greatly influence the moral take-home message for audiences.

Future opportunities for science fiction to contribute to bioethics

There is scope for science fiction to continue to play a major role in shaping public education and opinion on bioethical matters, while avoiding the overly negative representations commonly seen in this relationship. Some may even argue there is a responsibility to provide alternatives in bioethics literature for the purely dystopian images of scientific advancement so often seen in texts like *Frankenstein*, *Brave New World* and *Gattaca*. Not all uses of science fiction in bioethics need to be negatively motivated, as these speculative fictions also have the potential to promote accessible public debate concerning the possible benefits of emerging reproductive biotechnologies. For example, Bujold's Vorkosigan Saga, set in a world in which IVF and ectogenesis have replaced biological gestation, represents a mostly positive alternative to Huxley's dystopia. While references to this text can be found within the realm of disability studies, due to the presence of a disabled protagonist, it is almost entirely absent from the bioethical literature concerning ectogenesis. Bujold's complex treatment of reproductive biotechnologies and their associated ethical and political concerns is more balanced than Huxley's, demonstrating both the pros and cons of technological intervention in human reproduction.

H. Bruce Franklin defines science fiction as 'the literature which, growing with science and technology, evaluates it and relates it meaningfully to the rest of human existence'.[104] This highlights the future of science fiction as a medium for the negotiation of science into society, bridging the two 'gaps' both Csicsery-Ronay Jr. and Eugene Thacker identify: the 'technical gap' between what can be conceived in the imagination and that which is currently available, and the 'ethico-political gap' between what *could* become possible and what *should* be allowed to occur in the future.[105] This relies on science fiction authors continuing to anticipate future possible worlds, in which issues like posthuman citizenship, clone rights and the reproductive liberty of the genetically enhanced are being actively debated. Just as Jameson defends the special relationship between science fiction and social development,[106] Csicsery-Ronay Jr. believes the genre serves as a 'mode of awareness' of the scientific world, existing between the poles of imagination and realization of 'scientific-technological transformations'.[107] However, as discussed throughout this chapter, within bioethics scholarship, science fiction is currently being exploited almost exclusively to promote socially conservative political agendas.

There are examples of positive representations of reproductive biotechnologies to be found in science fiction, which could be used to argue in favour of technological development. Hamilton's concerns about the public relations issue facing many areas of biotechnology perhaps go some way toward explaining why this opportunity is rarely taken advantage of in practice.[108] One obvious barrier relates to accuracy, as fiction authors and filmmakers are focused on entertaining, rather than educating. For example, Kirby notes that while in the real world human genetic engineering is most commonly employed to correct life-threatening genetic conditions, science fiction stories 'rarely feature this as a plot element because it does not make for an action-packed narrative'.[109] Eutopian narratives (depicting idealized worlds) also suffer this disadvantage, with Jameson claiming they will always elicit the 'stirrings of a fear ... the fear of boredom'.[110] While certainly under-represented in the genre, there have been a number of successful science fiction stories that have characterized reproductive biotechnologies and alternative methods of procreation in a positive light, contributing to the creation of an ideal world. For example, Piercy's *Woman on the Edge of Time* (1976) depicts a fictional society in which ectogenesis has brought about total sexual equality; similarly, Le Guin's *The Left Hand of Darkness* (1969) explores an alien society in which fixed gender distinctions do not exist; thus, the burdens of reproduction fall equally across all members of the population.[111] The fact that these texts are comparatively overlooked in bioethical literature exposes the dominant conservatism behind the use of science fiction language and imagery in bioethical debate. This is especially the case when considering that the technologies or social norms facilitating more equal contributions to human reproduction form part (or all) of the fictional novum for these texts, which, as demonstrated above, is not the case for the more frequently cited *Brave New World*. Ectogenesis is incidental to Huxley's plot but essential for Piercy's.

In her analysis of science fiction's potential to assist in comprehending 'new biopolitical subjectivities', Squier claims the genre is now 'only a grim commentary on life as we must live it; no longer fantasy, but documentary'.[112] Given the pervasiveness of dystopia in the genre, if true, this is bleak news indeed. However, an alternative perspective would allow science fiction narratives to serve as a tool to shape possible futures. Lyman Tower Sargent claims utopia 'is at the root of all radicalism ... the archetype and harbinger of social change', and that visions of the future can have a tangible effect on social and political realities.[113] Thus, Mulford Q. Sibley notes that utopian science fiction has both persuasive and subversive power, fostering an interest in 'social questions' among readers and providing a palatable form of political instruction.[114] Redressing the under-utilization of science-fictional references to also promote liberal, pro-technological political agendas represents an opportunity for science fiction to be engaged in more balanced discussions of future reproductive biotechnologies.

Necessarily concerned with the socio-political aspects of an altered world, science fictions – and particularly utopian narratives – yield a rich source of hypotheticals for bioethicists to explore. Ideas and images from science fiction texts feature prominently in many bioethical debates, particularly those connected with the artificial creation or manipulation of human life. This demonstrates that science fiction authors may be in a unique position to influence public opinion in these areas by providing a common language to mediate between scientists and the public and producing fictional 'worlds of reference' for bioethics to explore. As an exploration of the scientific imaginary, science fiction has a distinct role to play in biopolitics, but one that has only been fully exploited by one side of the technoscience political divide. As such, there exists an opportunity for engaging the public with more positive representations of future reproductive biotechnologies, including cloning, ectogenesis and genetic engineering. The use of science fiction language in bioethics highlights an opportunity for the genre to be involved with the re-enchantment of science and technology while also bearing a social responsibility for providing meaningful philosophical and political debates on the potential impact of emerging technologies on society. The final chapter will suggest some methods by which these opportunities and duties might be approached.

5

Things to do with (science fiction) stories

When it comes to narrative ethics, Nelson asks: 'Do bedtime stories mold character? Do movies and plays install or shift a society's ethical norms? … And, if narratives do inform the moral life … *ought* they so to inform it?'[1] This final chapter will posit that the answer to these questions is the quintessential bioethicist response: *it depends*. Fictional narratives can shape ethical understanding (and misunderstanding), but this does not guarantee that they will. Nevertheless, there is a case to be made that, where moral influence is expected, responsible use can and should be the norm when introducing science fiction texts into bioethical debate. Returning to Nelson's five things to do with stories – namely, read, tell, compare, conduct literary analysis and invoke them – this chapter will focus on the fourth item: employing tools of literary analysis to explore the ethical dimensions of science fiction narratives depicting ectogenesis. In so doing, it aims to demonstrate a more meaningful engagement between the narrative genres of science fiction and bioethics than the scaremongering often seen in the previous chapter. Following Lomotey-Nakon and Lanphier's recommendation, the major case study to be considered here is Butler's *Dawn* (1987), the first book of the Xenogenesis trilogy. This is a particularly appropriate text, given that it considers the technology of interest while also providing a critique of the liberal feminist perspective adopted in this book.

This chapter will open with a brief description of bioethics-in-literature methodology before considering literary and narratological interpretations of Butler's work. It will then consider how science fiction images from some of the other texts considered in this book could contribute to discussions of design ethics for the artificial womb, before drawing all these elements together to propose a method of incorporating science fiction into a mode of anticipatory ethics for emerging technologies, including ectogenesis.

Bioethics-in-literature

At the most fundamental level, both ethics and literature describe actions and their consequences, often with some evaluative purpose. As such, Catherine Belling claims, 'bioethics – as the negotiation of right choices in biomedical science, health-care policy, and clinical practice – is inextricably entangled with fiction – the imaginative exploration of the possible consequences of human choices'.[2] The bioethics-in-literature approach exploits this relationship, allowing stories to fill in the context that philosophical thought experiments often painstakingly remove. When considering Terry and Williams' account of the methodology, Brody states:

> According to Terry and Williams, real-life events and descriptions of these events are fraught with ambiguity, and it is the job of the ethical analysis patiently to strip away the various levels of ambiguity until what remains is amenable to being understood in terms of agreed-upon ethical concepts and principles. By contrast, literature thrives on ambiguity, and coming to understand a work of literature often means coming to see ambiguity where none was seen before. Ethics, it seems, wants us to see face to face, while literature bids us peer through a glass, darkly .... If this is so, then we will have to set aside the most fundamental objectives of the bioethics course if we want to do justice to the literary works we bring into it.[3]

He compares this to the principlist approach to teaching and doing bioethics, where instead of being a potential source of new ethical knowledge, case studies represent 'rather the instantiation of more general concepts and principles'.[4] Such an approach may, for example, use narratives simply as a way of exploring the traditional four pillars of Western biomedical ethics – autonomy, beneficence, non-maleficence and justice – without questioning whether these principles are the most important elements to consider in the given scenario. For Howard Braswell, this is tantamount to placing these very bioethical principles and protocols above scrutiny, rather than allowing fictional explorations to challenge the common assumptions of the field.[5] Brody further claims such practices treat essential literary elements, such as a character's motives or intentions, as irrelevant to moral decision-making, despite the fact that ethical dilemmas also exist within specific socio-cultural contexts that have their own histories and 'narrative meaning'.[6] Ultimately, he concludes that using fiction in bioethical instruction while failing to engage with its ambiguities 'would not simply be an example of bad literary criticism. It would be incomplete bioethics'.[7] This criticism would seem to apply to several of the uses of science fiction described in the previous chapter but is diametrically opposed to how the bioethics-in-literature approach is intended to function. Instead of stripping back layers of complexity in search of a universal principle for action guidance, this method embraces the contradictions and conflicts between different subjectivities. As Christina Bieber Lake puts it: 'contrary to conventional wisdom, moral reasoning is less dependent on laws or principles than it is on metaphorical concepts'.[8] As noted in the previous chapter, science fiction provides a vast wealth of metaphors for bioethicists and the public to draw on.

With respect to using science fiction narratives for bioethics-in-literature analyses, Eric S. Rabkin posits:

> Science fiction, the literature defined by its concern for the possibilities and social implications of scientific and technological change, provides a dramatic mirror for bioethics. … In as much as ethics reflects both the character of individuals and that of groups, making bioethical judgments requires examining diverse individual characters in diverse relations to groups. Science fiction runs these human thought experiments for us.[9]

Thus, context, individual characterization and interpersonal relationships become central, rather than dismissible, parts of the process of bioethical reflection, knowledge acquisition and evaluation. This expands, rather than limits, the potential of these stories to develop the moral imagination. Science fiction narratives can make bioethical dilemmas 'come alive' in the same way author Joan Slonczewski claims *Star Trek*'s perpetually reproducing 'tribbles' can help students in non-science disciplines consider the ramifications of overpopulation.[10] Noting a scientist could 'extrapolate at will from the exponential growth of bacteria to an exploding population of humans', Slonczewski claims others are 'less likely to make that leap', requiring some form of mediation for this knowledge.[11] As previously discussed, science fiction has become one such mediator, potentially serving as a substitute when other forms of experiential knowledge are lacking. For bioethics, exploring the consequences of emerging technologies on different individuals and populations possessing full back stories and social networks allows for a degree of perspective-taking that might be difficult to access otherwise. These fictional characters can then replace the archetypal patient, next-of-kin, physician, etc., from the two-dimensional clinical vignettes of the bioethics classroom.

This section will now consider some examples of bioethics-in-literature analyses from different cultural perspectives. The first is Belling's discussion of the film *Coma* (1978) and the 1977 novel it was based on of the same name. While these texts are considered medical thrillers, they possess various characteristics of the science fiction genre as well. Focused on US and UK audiences' responses to these texts, Belling relates interviews and studies demonstrating that the negative depictions of doctors killing their patients to harvest and sell their organs in *Coma*, influenced some people to refuse organ donation in the real world.[12] She claims the film effectively manifested the 'moral horror' of 'instrumentalizing a patient', feeding into a growing distrust of medical professionals and their increasing use of biotechnologies with the power to blur the boundaries between life and death.[13] With regard to new life-support systems that could sustain brain-dead patients, she notes:

> Both bioethics and medical suspense fiction were responses to the radical epistemological and moral instability caused by biotechnology's new abilities to modify human life and death, and to socio-cultural changes opening those questions to increasingly active input from the public. The academic response to this crisis was the discipline of bioethics; its necessary popular corollary was the medical thriller.[14]

Thus, Belling claims, 'public bioethics' is that which occurs 'in the imagination that feeds on bestsellers and television', and that ethicists should not underestimate the persuasive power of these popular narratives.[15] Understanding this locus of bioethical inquiry, therefore, requires close engagement with these sources of data. This should not be cursory or dismissive, but rather capitalize on the depth of analysis available when considering the narratives as a whole.

On the same topic of transplant medicine, Kaori Sasaki considers the influence of Japanese science fiction manga and anime on organ donation protocols in Japan.[16] She claims that the 'major bioethical topics in Japan' were 'mapped out' in science fiction, and 'sci-fi narratives played a key role in formulating and circulating social attitudes toward bioethics' in the country.[17] Naming robotics and nuclear power as two fields of science and technology that bring up various ethical issues for the population, Sasaki observes:

> With robots, earlier studies indicated that the Japanese sci-fi manga (漫画) and anime (アニメ) genres have influenced the Japanese development of robot technologies and the associated public expectations. ... In contrast, numerous researchers have discussed how Japanese sci-fi representations of nuclear power have produced skeptical and critical attitudes among Japanese citizens. ... sci-fi imaginations and bioethical queries are interwoven within Japanese society.[18]

According to Sasaki, science-fictional robots played a role in how Japanese organ transplant law developed, suggesting that the treatment of donation after brain death relied on a 'sci-fi motif, originating in the Japanese manga genre' that exemplified Jean Baudrillard's concept of the 'symbolic exchange of life and death'.[19] She elaborates:

> The motif is basically composed of a provision of deathbed care by a marginal being (e.g., an android) to a human being and an exchange of body parts or functions (e.g., an organ) between them through which the existential value of life and death is mutually appreciated and blessed.[20]

This motif, she claims, was applied to the issue of organ donation after brain death and became 'embodied' in the Organ Transplantation Act of 1997.[21] But more importantly, it had already been woven into the discourse of the 'brain-death problem' in Japanese society as distinct from Western biomedical accounts of the phenomenon and its implications for transplant medicine.[22] The exploration of existential crises for androids in science fiction was incorporated into discussions regarding the ambiguous moral status of brain-dead individuals, exemplifying how the bioethics-in-literature methodology can be deployed in cases of ontological uncertainty. Sasaki notes that for androids, this existential confusion can be due to 'the *addition* of body parts to a human body or the absolute *lack* of a human biological mechanism', thereby allowing characters like *Ghost in the Shell*'s (1989–2003) Major Motoko Kusanagi to articulate 'a distinctive bioethical query on ontology in connection with body-parts/function exchange between life and death' that is immediately relevant to the brain-dead organ donor scenario.[23] The potential to apply this reasoning regarding humanness and its relationship to specific biological functions to discussions of ectogenesis, both from the perspective of the artificially gestated and the mothers who will not be physically pregnant, should be apparent.

As a brief final case, Nicola Gavioli considers the impact of literature on concepts of euthanasia ethics in Brazil, claiming fiction can complicate 'binary thinking of acceptance or refusal of euthanasia' by considering the 'singularity of each situation' and the people involved.[24] Again, this is the opposite of stripping down the narrative in search of core, universal principles and, like in the previous case, may be assisted by the fact that these audiences are not beholden to the dominant Western principlist ethics paradigm. Claiming fiction can be more nuanced than the politically motivated journalistic accounts of end-of-life decisions, Gavioli suggests:

> Works of literature, reports, and *crönicas* [chronicles] that interrogate, provoke, and challenge the political and public silence on euthanasia, assisted suicide, and living wills, are per se examples of activist writing, no matter the position defended by their authors.[25]

Thus, fictional authors are doing the imaginative work of bioethics when others fail to deliver this. However, if debate is lacking elsewhere, the position an author takes may be more influential than anticipated, of which Nelson warns: 'If, then, we find our imaginations gripped by a story whose moral resources are lopsided or too narrowly confined to one ethical point of view, we will get from it very little guidance'.[26] The science fiction author may well defend any bias in their work as serving literary entertainment goals, rather than promoting balanced bioethical debate, leaving the onus on those who invoke these narratives to use them appropriately. The next section will consider one potential way of promoting this agenda: applying tools of literary analysis to the use of science fiction in bioethics.

Literary analysis and interpretation

Much like in the sciences, literary analysis involves focusing on a topic or specific research question, gathering and interpreting evidence (in this case, textual evidence) and drawing conclusions on the basis of this evidence. These conclusions are often concerned with elucidating the meaning of the text (or parts thereof) or serve to defend a particular argument regarding the plot, characters, setting, imagery, etc. Employing tools of literary analysis and interpretation can thus form part of a bioethics-in-literature approach, with the specific topic of interest typically being an ethical question or treatment of a scientific or technological innovation. However, even within literary studies, these techniques – and particularly narratology, as will be considered in the next section – are often reserved for 'capital-L' literature, rather than popular texts. This is despite the fact that, as Belling notes, '[p]opular fiction responds to, and may exacerbate, public anxieties in ways that more highbrow literary texts may not'.[27] As demonstrated in previous chapters, for emerging biotechnologies, it is often science fiction, rather than classical or literary fiction, that provides the most fertile ground for cultivating bioethical discussions. Nevertheless, in her article, 'The Art of Medicine: Cognitive Estrangement, Science Fiction and Medical Ethics', Priscilla Wald claims that when it comes to defining what is human:

> The field of medical humanities has long turned to realist fiction to help address such ethical questions. Yet few commentators have explored the perspective on those questions offered by the (often debased) genre of science fiction. The fantastic, futuristic, and often alien settings that are conventions of the genre lend themselves to broad speculation about the boundaries between what is and what is not human. Furthermore, the strangeness of these settings enfranchises speculation since it does not reproduce readers' preconceived ideas about present-day social issues with which they believe they identify.[28]

In the absence of careful literary analysis and close textual reading though, the sensationalist uses of science fiction in bioethics seen in the previous chapter will persist unchallenged. On the flip side, even when handling dystopian narratives, balanced debate is possible if texts are considered within their broader contexts and subjected to rigorous analysis. As such, a study of the representation of ectogenesis in science fiction can include references to the unique world-building and societal structures created in the narrative, and not just the raw imagery connected with the technology or its association with any negative socio-cultural outcomes, including the recurrent themes covered in Chapter 3. It can also speculate on what changes to the above elements might materially alter how the technology *could* function in the fictional universe, for example, how ectogenesis might be viewed differently in Huxley's text if isolated from both the 'Bokanovsky's Process' for human cloning and the totalitarian governance structure of the World State.[29] In this way, the overly simplistic logic that suggests that since *Brave New World* is a dystopia and happens to contain ectogenesis, that ectogenesis is therefore necessarily dystopian, can be interrogated and rejected.

Zimmerman claims that for new reproductive biotechnologies to enhance women's lives, they need to 'gain political and financial control' over their development and implementation.[30] Fictional utopias represent one method of teasing out how such control may be seized. She continues:

> Artificial insemination. Sperm banks. *Ex utero* fertilization (test tube babies). Surrogate mothers. Genetic screening. Amniocentesis. *In vitro* fetal development (artificial wombs). The words rocket out from science fiction fantasy to the borders of reality, and they are rocketing at speeds faster than the ethical light it takes to comprehend them.[31]

This exposes one of the major impediments to enhancing the relationship between bioethics and science fiction through using in-depth literary analysis – close textual analysis *takes time*. For works of fiction to genuinely help explore bioethical issues means taking the time to let the 'ethical light' of the story penetrate the fog of uncertainty, without simply trying to eradicate the narrative ambiguities Brody considers essential to the practice of bioethics-in-literature.[32] The next two sections will introduce different aspects of one specific literary analysis tool to aid in this process – narratology – before applying both this and more general literary interpretative methods to exploring the representation of ectogenesis in Butler's *Dawn* (1987). This text has been chosen not only because it is an influential work of science fiction depicting many issues relevant to reproductive bioethics but also because it challenges the Anglo- and Eurocentric biases often present in similar works, while also highlighting how a liberal feminist agenda can fail to consider intersectional issues, such as racial discrimination.

Narratological analysis and point of view

According to Nelson, 'Perhaps the most significant ethical turn in literary criticism has been the emergence of the subfield of narratology, which developed out of structuralist linguistics'.[33] She notes that structuralism 'offered formal, scientific accounts of the grammar and deep structure of language, based on differences in sound production that could be marked, mapped, and classified', and that narratology assumed a similar methodology could be applied to 'folktales, films, and other narrative forms'.[34] Instead of primarily focusing on interpretation, narratology considers the structural elements of narratives.

For narratologist, Gerald Prince, 'any narrative is the representation of real or fictive situations and events in a time sequence'.[35] Wolf Schmid goes further to suggest that an intrinsic property of all narratives is that they also depict 'at least one change of state' during the narrative timeline, whether that be in a person, or the external circumstances being described.[36] For a bioethics case study, some example 'changes of state' might include pregnancy, illness or death, or being eligible to receive a treatment allocation versus being denied. Decisions made along the way by different stakeholders all contribute to the outcome state. In the first instance, met contraceptive need, access to fertility assistance and preservation, access to safe and legal abortion, and the availability of quality maternal healthcare practices will influence the pregnant/not pregnant state. For life and death issues, relevant bioethical considerations might include the right to refuse lifesaving interventions (cf Dax Cowart), appropriate methods of resolving disagreements regarding the care of incapacitated patients (cf Terri Schiavo), the impact of 'do not resuscitate' orders and advanced care directives, age-based resource allocation protocols and different types of triages (e.g., standard or disaster/combat triage), the dead donor rule regarding eligibility to become an organ donor (cf Sasaki's study above) and many more. When these dilemmas are narrativized into a bioethics case study, the same rules of literary and narratological analysis can be applied to understanding them. When they are brought to life in fiction, bioethical analysis can similarly shed light on their ethical meaning.

For Prince, one of the most significant goals for the field of narratology is discovering an explanation for the phenomenon of 'narrative competence':

> not only do we all have certain intuitions (or know certain rules) about the nature of narratives and what they mean, but also, to a certain extent at least, we all have the same intuitions and know the same rules. It is this set of rules and intuitions, this narrative competence, that allows us (human beings) to produce and process narratives, to tell, retell, paraphrase, expand, summarize, and understand them in like manner. Narratology studies the form and functioning of narrative and tries to account for narrative competence. More specifically, it examines what all narratives have in common.[37]

These elements in common are typically referred to in narrative studies as the 'triadic set' of fabula, story (or syuzhet, сюжет) and text.[38] The fabula represents a sequence of events and transitions following a cause-and-effect logical chronology, the story is how this raw data has been re-organized and presented in a particular order, and the text refers to the signs – e.g., words on the page or shots of a film – communicating these other aspects from a narrator to a narratee.[39] This narrative exchange can be further complicated by considering the roles of the actual or implied author and the actual or implied audience involved. In terms of Prince's idea of 'narrative competence', a relationship can also be seen with Delany's claims about consumers of science fiction being primed to read texts in a particular way, following additional narrative 'rules' specific to the genre's conventions, as discussed in Chapter 2.[40] David Herman suggests that postclassical narratology should thus consider how audiences are able to 'activate relevant kinds of knowledge with or without explicit textual cues to guide them', suggesting narrative forms can exploit this process of knowledge activation to 'privilege some world models over others'.[41] Personally identifying with a protagonist or situation represents one way authors can elicit sympathy from readers for specific characters and their world views.

While a lot of narratology has focused on classical literature, in his book, *Film Narratology*, Peter Verstraten argues that the same structural features also exist in movies. Instead of printed words, he says the filmic text 'consists of a series of moving images on-screen that are (usually) accompanied by sound', the fabula remains the same, while the story still represents 'the specific way in which plot elements are ordered'.[42] Of David Bordwell's account of film narrative, Verstraten states: 'For Bordwell, a narratological analysis revolves around the interaction between narrative tactics and stylistic features', claiming this is 'analogous to the more familiar distinction between content and form'.[43] In 'Three Dimensions of Film Narrative', Bordwell further describes some of these stylistic choices by filmmakers as 'presentational tactics', aimed at shaping what information the audience receives.[44] This is similar to Hellsten's claim described in the previous chapter, regarding the potential for fictional accounts of new technologies to push certain ethical issues 'out of focus'.[45]As such, Verstraten posits 'narrativity in cinema is created by an interaction between the narrative agent and the viewer'.[46] What is important here is that this interaction is heavily mediated, with certain interpretations of the text being more favourably supported than others. Tilmann Köppe and Tom Kindt describe this phenomenon noting, '[f]ictional texts can authorize (virtually) all kinds of imaginings'.[47] What is also implied in these two statements though is that some stories and storytellers may be privileged over others, while some types of imagining may be suppressed. This may go some way to accounting for the poverty of imagination seen in science fiction and the bioethics literature that engages with it regarding the potential for ectogenesis to promote sexual equality in human reproduction, as discussed in the Introduction. It also introduces the major aspect of narratology to be considered here: point of view. Although there are many narratological elements that are worth considering when bringing science fiction into bioethics (characterization, setting, rhythm, frequency, etc.), given the time constraints discussed in the previous section, analysing the significance of who is given a voice in the narratives invoked seems like a reasonable minimum standard to demand.

In his article, 'Documentary Bioethics: Visual Narratives for Generations X and Y', John C. Stys claims: 'Narrative can be defined rather simply as a story or the telling of story'.[48] However, a story is a thing, whereas the telling of a story is an action. This distinction can be very significant when narratives are brought into bioethics, as only some characters (real and imagined) are given the privileged position of storyteller. This is something Nelson comments on when reflecting on her time as associate editor of the *Hastings Center Report*, where she recalls the case studies she would review 'were tales told almost exclusively by physicians, or, occasionally, by other health care workers … told in such a way as to drive the reader toward a particular ethical conclusion'.[49] The point of view of other 'characters' in the stories, including patients and their families, was largely absent.

In narratology, 'point of view' as introduced by Henry James in 'The Art of Fiction' (1884) highlights how stories are told from a particular perspective, dictating the angle from which the tale is explored.[50] Gérard Genette later suggested traditional accounts of point of view failed to distinguish between whose perspective was being adopted and who was narrating the story, summarizing the 'three-term typology' that arose in modal narratology as: *Narrator > Character*, an omniscient narrator who tells more than the characters know (possessing Jean Pouillon's 'vision from behind'); *Narrator = Character*, a narrator limited to the knowledge of the specific character narrating the story (possessing Georges Blin's 'restricted field' of knowledge, or Pouillon's 'vision with') and *Narrator < Character*, a narrator that provides less information than the character has (Pouillon's 'vision from without').[51] Genette coined the term 'focalization' to remove this confusion between 'who speaks' and 'who sees'[52] and to 'avoid the too specifically visual connotations of the terms *vision*, *field*, and *point of view*'.[53] The ocularcentrism of early theories of imagination discussed in Chapter 2 is thus relevant again when considering structuralist accounts of narrative. For Genette, the omniscient narrator represents zero focalization (the knowledge conveyed to the audience is not restricted by the adopted perspective); the character as narrator represents internal focalization (allowing the audience insights into the character's thoughts, mood and emotions, but limiting access to information according to the character's own level of knowledge or bias); and finally, external focalization refers to when the narrator can only convey the external actions of the characters (without access to their 'thoughts or feelings').[54] As such, Sabine Schlickers claims focalization can be considered 'the knowledge of the narrator in relation to the characters', providing the examples of an intradiegetic narrator (a narrator existing within the fictional world) and an extradiegetic narrator (e.g., an external voiceover in a documentary), with the latter often appearing more trustworthy and knowledgeable.[55]

Schmid criticizes Genette's reimagining of point of view, suggesting it 'reduces the complex phenomenon … to a single feature, the mere restriction of knowledge'.[56] Nevertheless, whether focused on knowledge, emotion, action or subjective perception, point of view and focalization are useful tools for analysing bioethical narratives. They are also related to the concept of narrative voice, a series of stylistic choices including whether the text is written in the first- (I/we), second- (you) or third-person (she/he/they). To demonstrate the significance of these, compare an omniscient narrator stating 'the patient was in pain' to a physician character narrating the same, but as an evaluative judgement that they have made themselves. The former is providing a narrated fact, whereas the latter may represent what Wayne C. Booth labels an 'unreliable narrator', one who knowingly or unknowingly misleads the audience due to their own lack of knowledge or self-awareness.[57] Compare again to an externally focalized account, 'the patient flinched', or a first-person narration from the patient themselves, where they state 'it hurt'. This last example directly connects to how fiction can develop the moral emotions, by providing what Schmid describes as 'direct access into other people's inner worlds'.[58] He continues:

> The natural staging of someone else's inner world is certainly one of the reasons for the anthropological and cultural significance of fiction. The reader can step outside of himself or herself and not only lead someone else's life but slip into someone else's subjectivity and tentatively play out someone else's perceptions and ambitions. No conversation and no psychological document can offer so much alterity. Only immersion in the inner world of the fictive other gives a person the possibility of forming a notion of his or her own identity.[59]

This recognizes the importance of exploring different subjectivities and the significance of considering which voices are deemed authoritative in any given narrative. When addressing a phenomenon like pregnancy, where great diversity in experience and perception exists and the majority of people in positions of social authority have no access to direct experience, who is allowed to tell stories and construct meaning is important. In 'The Pregnant Imagination, Fetal Rights, and Women's Bodies', Julia Epstein recounts how maternal testimony has been replaced by medical authority when determining fundamental aspects of pregnancy, echoing Duden's study described in Chapter 2.[60] Epstein similarly notes that in the eighteenth century, '[a] pregnancy did not exist until there was a quickening, as announced by the pregnant woman, and a child did not exist until it was born alive'.[61] She suggests that shifting views of pregnancy and women's bodily autonomy in the present means that 'female *interiority* has been made public, while women's bodily *exterior* has attained juridical and moral privacy rights'.[62] In other words, women's utterances have been replaced by ultrasound images, exposing their interior wombs while denying their interior worlds. Narratives that exclusively adopt the point of view of foetuses or future children born using reproductive biotechnologies also work to silence women's voices as an authoritative source of meaning regarding procreation. This also shows that narratives often do not just have an informational and/or emotional point of view, but a moral one as well.

The moral of the story and feminist narratology

In 'Gender and Narratology', Marion Gymnich claims: 'the textual arrangement of focaliser(s) and narrative voice(s) may challenge existing power structures by privileging the perspectives and voices of those narrators/characters whose views tend to be neglected in public discourses in a particular cultural context'.[63] For a bioethics case study, this might involve seeking out narrative perspectives that challenge clinical hierarchies and promote diverse voices. As Pritha Kundu notes: 'According to the Foucauldian scheme, clinical authority, like religion or state-laws, has a controlling power over what is considered normative, sane, orderly, and proper'.[64] In healthcare in general, this has led to the classification of some patients as non-compliant or difficult when they do not conform to the roles assigned to them or follow the directions of medical experts. When it comes to human reproduction, this bias has contributed to the over-medicalization of pregnancy and childbirth and the devaluation of women's lived experiences and testimonies. When outlining the components of stories, Nelson notes that 'stories constitute people's *identities*, and so give rise to normative expectations for behavior', and that using stories as paradigm ethical cases (as defended by proponents of casuistry) suggests there are 'shared moral understandings that are already embedded in our actual practices' that can guide actions in the present.[65] However, she reiterates that stories are *depictive*, only representative of certain actions; *connective*, in that they assume specific causal relationships and intertextual associations; *selective*, choosing only to cover elements the teller finds pertinent and *interpretive*, determining the meaning by choosing what actions are included and in what sequence.[66] As such, the elevation of foetal interests as coinciding with the silencing of women's voices regarding experiences of gestation, coupled with increasing state interference and social policing of pregnant women's bodies and behaviours, requires powerful counter-narratives and alternative normative judgements to allow for serious consideration of the liberating potential of emerging reproductive biotechnologies, including ectogenesis. If using fiction in place of traditional case studies, the same opportunities for inclusive practice arise, dictating that a range of perspectives be included.

For Stys, '[w]hen one discusses any use of narrative, it is important to mention some of the inevitable moral issues that arise', claiming that first and foremost, this includes reflecting on who is given a platform to tell their story and what their agenda may be.[67] For the medical professionals providing the case studies Nelson commented on, various motivations may be implied, but by obscuring the subjectivity of the 'narrator', such accounts assume the guise of omniscience while still being thoroughly enmeshed in the personal context of a specific 'character' involved. That this character already possesses authority in the situation further alienates the perspectives of others in the narrative. In *The Moral Laboratory*, Jémeljan Hakemulder highlights some important consequences of this when discussing the results of a systematic study into using literature for moral instruction:

> In general, the data show that literature-based treatments have effects on readers' attitudes, norms, values, beliefs, self-concept, social abilities, and level of critical and moral thinking. Besides positive effects, the researchers also assessed negatives ones. Reading stories with unfavorable portrayals of some outgroup caused negative attitudes toward that group.[68]

Noting that 'many educators believe that narratives can be more effective instruments in teaching moral lessons than philosophical treatises', Hakemulder claims fiction can enhance the ability to draw 'psychological inferences about the emotions, thoughts, and motives others have in certain situations', inducing an emotional and 'pre-ethical' effect.[69] Converting this into an ethical encounter with otherness requires an appreciation of both the structure and context of storytelling, particularly if focused on the highly gendered phenomenon of procreation. For some, this has led to a call for a feminist narratology that takes gender equity issues into account in narratological analysis.

At the outset, speaking of a feminist narratology seems oxymoronic, as structuralist accounts aimed to analyse texts based on formal characteristics alone, or, as Gymnich puts it, 'without referring to gender (or any other social or cultural categories for that matter)'.[70] However, it is not just the point of view or focalization that is relevant when encountering a text but also whether the perspectives or focalizers are rendered masculine or feminine.[71] As such, Gymnich notes that for pioneer feminist narratologist, Susan S. Lanser, gender became a 'category that is relevant to the analysis of the structural features of narratives'.[72] Lanser herself accuses classical narratology of suppressing the 'representational aspects of fiction' in favour of emphasizing the semiotic, claiming this is the opposite of what feminist critique attempts.[73] She argues her theory differs from

Genette's because it incorporates 'contextual approaches to meaning in narrative' rather than purely focusing on form.[74] This allows for the interrogation of how the different social status of various narrators and focalizers impacts audience receptivity and value for the message conveyed.[75] For Lanser, this is a question of audience trust and affection for the speaker in a narrative and relates to that speaker's stance, in other words, their relationship to the message.[76] She claims: 'a given stance and its phraseological form can affect the very substance of what is said' and not just how it is interpreted.[77] The following case study will adopt the position that gender is an important consideration in both literary interpretation and narratological analysis, particularly when focusing on reproductive technologies. Thus, the power imbalances seen between physicians and patients in bioethical case studies and fictional representations of healthcare narratives can also be exacerbated by other features, including age, gender, sexuality, socio-economic status, education level and many other characteristics.

Case study: Octavia E. Butler's *Dawn* (1987)

On the surface, Butler's *Dawn* may seem an odd choice to focus on when exploring science-fictional representations of ectogenesis; after all, artificial wombs are only explicitly mentioned once in the text. However, it contains elements of all the science fiction tropes typically associated with ectogenesis discussed in Chapter 3, which cause horror for the humans in the narrative precisely because ectogenesis is rejected as a possible solution by their alien captors. In this story, Earth was rendered uninhabitable by nuclear war, and the few human survivors were captured by an alien species that kept them in suspended animation for 250 years while intermittently conducting experiments on them. Although there is no single 'mad scientist', the experiments described demonstrate a complete lack of concern for the human subjects, feeding into what Irene Sanz Alonso considers the main ethical issue dramatized in the narrative: lack of consent.[78] This alien species consists of male and female Oankali, and the sexless ooloi, who control the species' reproduction through rearranging the genetic elements of offspring. The males and females of each reproductive unit are typically close relatives (often siblings) and cannot reproduce without an ooloi, who guarantees no negative genetic effects from these consanguineous unions.[79] The species is also evolutionarily driven to crossbreed with aliens, incorporating their genetic information to create hybrids. As the Oankali retain the genetic memory of previous crossbreeds, the narrative outlines a future of animal-alien-human hybrids, touching on both the hybrid tropes considered in Chapter 3. It is also clearly an example of the genetic manipulation and human augmentation tropes, with the aliens constantly defending their genetic experimentation by claiming the resultant offspring will have superior abilities.

When it comes to the human farming trope, due to the small original sample population available, the Oankali actively farm the human survivors in order to better study them. There are various breeding stock metaphors used throughout the text, including 'human crop'[80] and 'captive breeders', with comparisons drawn to species preservation programs humans currently engage in for endangered animal species.[81] The Oankali's human breeding program is facilitated by several reproductive technologies, including artificial insemination, surrogacy, cloning and ectogenesis, with the latter considered necessary because relying on biological pregnancies could not produce enough humans to study, due to the lack of available wombs. Fulfilling another trope, the Oankali's way of life, including their 'gene trading' reproductive model, is necessary to sustain their space colonization efforts, with certain characters noting they must continue to travel and merge with more species for their survival. Finally, the constant threat of involuntary genetic parenthood permeates the narrative and is directly linked to the issue of sexual inequality and reproductive coercion.

The book opens at the point in the plot timeline where the Oankali intend to implement their long-term species crossbreeding program using human biological pregnancies, rather than the laboratory experiments they have been conducting for over two centuries. This involves genetic modification of the human male and female survivors and facilitating the creation of Oankali-human-ooloi embryos. The impact of the modifications means the humans are rendered otherwise infertile. To secure the cooperation of the survivors, the Oankali select a human liaison, Lilith Iyapo, whom they train to cohabitate with Oankali and ooloi. Lilith's role is to prepare the other humans for the 'gene trade' by incrementally increasing the number released from suspended animation and building them into a collective. She is also tasked with training them to live on the rehabilitated Earth, which, as the Oankali do not trust the species not to destroy itself a second time, will require them to 'begin again' – for example, adapt to life in the forest with no provided technology.[82] The aliens tell Lilith they have even gone so far as to destroy any ruins from previous human civilizations they found during their ecological restoration project, an act that devastates the former anthropologist.[83]

Throughout Lilith's enculturation into Oankali society, she undergoes various genetic modifications that allow her to interact with their semi-organic ship and grant her certain survival advantages, lest her human charges turn on her as a traitor. As such, Éva Federmayer claims *Dawn*:

> plays out the *Bildungsroman* of Lilith Iyapo. The narrative revolves around the changing of this young African American woman from an ordinary middle-class Human woman into a 'cyborg.' The extraterrestrial Oankali and their genetic engineers, the ooloi, accomplish this by augmenting her body, causing her to acquire enhanced physical and sensory capabilities that allow her to become a bridge between Humans and Oankali.[84]

The reliance on genetic modification to activate social and behavioural change is a persistent theme throughout the novel, often relying on essentialist views of what makes a human in general, and what makes a male or female human, in particular. As such, Nancy Jesser claims: 'Genetics is the science of Butler's science fiction. The translation of genotype into phenotype is the plot'.[85] In the case of Lilith and many of her 'brood' of awakened humans, the genetic manipulation of themselves and their offspring represents a violation, with Lilith claiming a hybrid child 'will be a thing–not human … it won't be human … that *is* what matters'.[86]

According to Jihun Yoo, works like Butler's *Dawn* and Margaret Atwood's *Oryx and Crake* (2003) 'explore genetic modification and the remaking of the human, and raise questions on the limits and ethics of science and technology'.[87] Yoo further claims:

> Of all literary genres, science and speculative fiction are perhaps most suitable to explore transhumanism and the posthuman condition in that they not only confound certain boundaries and binaries of Western culture but also reconfigure our notions about our current society and culture through the deployment of utopian, dystopian, and/or apocalyptic elements.[88]

Boundary violation is a recurrent theme in *Dawn*, including of gender roles and species boundaries. The text functions as a work of feminist literature because it challenges patriarchal assumptions, as well as racial stereotypes, providing an unfamiliar setting to discuss very familiar phenomena in the real world. Most importantly for Meghan Hurley-Powell, *Dawn* shows women's resistance to 'gender-based oppression in many ways and under the bleakest of circumstances'.[89] She claims that the feminist dystopian genre 'is impactful because it rejects the proverbial notion that obvious resistance strategies are more powerful than complex and nuanced resistance', suggesting Lilith's behaviour throughout *Dawn* is a good example of the latter.[90] Although she is forced to be compliant due to the power imbalance between her and her alien captors, she finds numerous ways to resist and rebel, ultimately training her awakened humans to '*Learn and run!*'[91]

While there are certainly elements of the cautionary tale present in *Dawn*, particularly regarding the development of genetic engineering technologies, Hurley-Powell claims the value of the 'feminist dystopian imagination … extends beyond scare tactics', suggesting Butler's work can contribute more than just a warning to women to fight against patriarchal powers to avoid Lilith's dystopian fate.[92] Returning to Sanz Alonso's claim that one of the primary ethical issues at stake in *Dawn* is consent,[93] by digging deeper than the surface horror motifs seen in many of the uses of science fiction demonstrated in the previous chapter, Butler's fictional world can yield alternative, pro-technological interpretations, including regarding the potential for ectogenesis to promote women's liberation.

Literary analysis and interpretation of *Dawn*

First employing thematic literary analysis, while the surface narrative of *Dawn* may be about post-apocalyptic futures, aliens and spaceships, the underlying message of the text concerns reproductive coercion in the real world and the violence of colonization. Rape and pregnancy are an ever-present threat throughout the story, with women's vulnerability to both readily on display. Most of the human female characters are almost raped (literally), while the entire survivor population is figuratively raped through the ooloi's interference in their sexual and reproductive lives. The ooloi's physical penetration of the human male and female couples, while neurologically stimulating sexual arousal and release, occurs without consent and often while the humans are drugged. One of the many heteronormative assumptions of the text is that this is more of a violation for the male characters, several of whom are spurred to violence in response. This is despite the fact that it is the women, including Lilith, who face forced, unwanted pregnancies as a result. Sanz Alonso notes:

> Science Fiction offers a whole different kind of literary analysis. Behind supernatural creatures, extraterrestrials, robots and other realities labelled as Science Fiction, we can discover how familiar SF situations are to us. Thus, we can find in SF literature something like a mirror of our own society, a mirror that is disguised through futuristic situations and discomforting worlds.[94]

From the Suvinian perspective, identifying and exploring the novum represent one of these new modes of literary analysis. In *Dawn*, the ooloi's genetic engineering has created the central innovation or 'fictional novelty' of Butler's text, which in turn has created a whole new method of rape – sexual coercion that goes all the way down to the nucleotides of human DNA.[95] Yoo describes the Oankali as 'rapacious hyper-exploiters of any organisms that they encounter ... [with] an inventive capacity to hide their exploitative intentions under the veneer of an eco-friendly method of living'.[96] The Oankali not only plan to colonize humanity's home planet but also to colonize the bodies of Earth's inhabitants as well. Yoo notes the fact that humans are given no other choice than to have their bodies used to 'cure' the Oankali's 'own evolutionary cul-de-sac', and occupy a subordinate position in relation to these aliens, bears 'a close resemblance to the relations between colonial rulers and subjects'.[97] In reproducing both sexual and racial inequality, Hurley-Powell claims Butler's text is 'rhetorically feminist', as it is emphasizing the same injustices in the real world while predicated on the ability of readers to identify the gendered power imbalances and how characters like Lilith subtly resist these.[98] She further notes that Lilith is often forced to be complicit because 'open and obvious resistance is impossible due to near constant surveillance', drawing attention to similar disempowering circumstances preventing open resistance to gender-based oppression in the real world.[99] Lilith must agree to become a 'reproductive vessel' and liaison for the Oankali or be returned to suspended animation forever.[100] If she cannot get the other humans to cooperate, Lilith might also die by their hands. As a challenge to liberal feminism, the text does not entertain the possibility that some women may be able to happily engage in this hybrid-species reproductive project without harming the interests of the others. All humans are at risk of annihilation through alien genomic contamination, and thus, all must learn to fight together to survive as a species.

For Justin Louis Mann, the constant association of reproductive capacity and death in *Dawn*, as well as the association of 'blackness, sexuality and subjection', frames the idea of human survival 'in terms of sexual vulnerability'.[101] He notes 'Lilith herself remains dubious of her ability to re-make the human social order without patriarchal white supremacy',[102] which seems to be confirmed in the narrative when Lilith reproduces sexual and racial violence against her human male partner, Joseph. Described as being a physically smaller, Asian man, Joseph is drugged when Lilith allows her ooloi partner, Nikanj, to penetrate them both, so she can experience 'an intimacy with Joseph that was beyond ordinary human experience'.[103] The following quote describes the encounter:

> She sandwiched Nikanj's body between her own and Joseph's, placing it for the first time in the ooloi position between two humans. For an instant that frightened her. This was the way she might someday be made pregnant with an other-than-human child.
>
> She felt it tremble against her and knew it was in.[104]

This is followed later by Lilith's consideration of Joseph's likely response:

> 'He might…' She forced herself to voice the thought. 'He might not want anything more to do with me when he realizes what I helped you do with him'.[105]

From the reader's perspective, this sexual experience was not something done *with* Joseph, but rather something done *to* him without consent. Even more problematically, future non-consensual encounters are justified by Nikanj by claiming Joseph's 'body has made a different choice' than his mind and 'words'[106]:

> 'The second time will be the hardest for you. I left you no choice the first time. You could not have understood what there was to choose. Now you have some small idea. And you have a choice.'
>
> He understood now. 'No!' he said sharply. 'Not again. … You said I could choose. I've made my choice!'[107]
>
> …
>
> 'Let go of me!'
>
> It smoothed its tentacles again. 'Be grateful, Joe. I'm not going to let go of you'.[108]

Even more disturbing is how this violation is described by the narrator:

> In a perverse way, Joseph too was probably enjoying himself, though he could not have said so.[109]
>
> …
>
> Now he was ready to accept what he had wanted from the beginning.[110]

Ironically, this manifestation of rape culture is positioned just before Lilith lectures the humans in her collective that 'There'll be no rape here!… Nobody here is property. Nobody here has the right to the use of anybody else's body. There'll be no back-to-the-Stone-Age, caveman bullshit!'[111] She does not address the possibility of a cave*woman* rapist using her superior strength and alien alliances to dominate a human male. Given all of Joseph's utterances vehemently refuse sexual consent, the description of him 'probably enjoying himself' is likely a product of the narrative being from Lilith's perspective, as will be considered later in this chapter. She has a vested interest in recasting this rape as something else because the alternative aligns her with the alien colonizers. As will also be demonstrated, it is Lilith's views on maternal medicine that impact how reproductive biotechnologies are treated in the text, and how future hybrid offspring are described: 'Medusa children. Snakes for hair. Nests of night crawlers for eyes and ears'.[112] This is also one of the many different references to ancient myth in the text.

Although there are various intertextual references throughout *Dawn* that are worthy of analysis, the connection of the protagonist to the mythology of Lilith is one of the more prevalent foci in literary scholarship. Michele Osherow notes that Butler's Lilith, like her namesake in rabbinic literature, becomes the 'incubator for a type of devil's spawn'.[113] She continues:

> In Butler's story, Lilith is not able to deny her reproductive strength. Her survival depends upon compliance, for it is through her biological potential for motherhood that Lilith maintains her place within the Oankali order. This is often the case with female aliens in science fiction. In this genre, particularly as it is reinscribed by women, the role of Mother is essential, representing the importance of a nurturing, life-giving force. …
>
> Highlighting Lilith as the mother of all reminds us, too, that Lilith is a mother, according to legend. She's not our mother, but she did give birth to armies of Lucifer's young. Her children are demons, but they are her children nonetheless, a facet of the story often overlooked by critics.[114]

Just as the Lilith of mythology was doomed to watch her demonic offspring die, so Butler's Lilith has already lost her husband and child and will stand guard as the rest of humanity's legacy is co-opted or destroyed. She cannot accept that humanity has survived its self-imposed apocalypse in any meaningful way unless its offspring remain fully human. That human children will be replaced by Oankali-human-ooloi hybrids, represents a reversal of how the mythical Lilith's offspring as Adam's first wife were replaced by the human offspring of Eve, as described in various midrashic texts. It is only by considering *Dawn* within the broader literary canon that such interpretations become available, and only through close textual analysis that additional bioethical issues come to light, as will now be demonstrated.

Bioethics and ectogenesis in *Dawn*

It is against the above backdrop of colonial horrors and reproductive coercion that a bioethical discussion of artificial gestation can be initiated. There are two relevant passages from *Dawn* to draw on here, although only one of them explicitly mentions artificial wombs. The first occurs when Lilith is introduced to another human who has been living with the Oankali, Paul Titus. Awakened when he was fourteen and kept isolated from other humans, Paul has been told by the Oankali that his 'genetic material has been used in over seventy children' in their breeding program.[115] He complains that despite this, he has 'never seen a woman' or been able to 'do it before', claiming the Oankali offered Lilith to him for sex if she was interested.[116] Lilith rejects him, having already said she has no intention of 'giving them a human child to tamper with',[117] to which Paul responded:

> 'You probably already have … They didn't have enough of us for what they call a normal trade … They had to make more'.
>
> 'While we slept? Somehow they – '
>
> 'Somehow!' he hissed. '*Anyhow!* They took stuff from men and women who didn't even know each other and put it together and made babies in women who never knew the mother or the father of their kid – and who maybe never got to know the kid. Or maybe they grew the baby in another kind of animal. They have animals they can adjust to – to incubate human fetuses, as they say. Or maybe they don't even worry about men and women. Maybe they just scrape some skin from one person and make babies out of it – cloning, you know … But if they've got one of you, they can use it to make another you even if you've been dead for a hundred years … They can make people in ways I don't even know how to talk about.'[118]

Paul later becomes violent and tries to rape Lilith.[119] It is after this encounter that she learns she has been involuntarily sterilized by the Oankali, although Nikanj assures her that when it is 'time for [her] to have children', this will be 'undone'.[120] Although the ooloi promises this will be according to Lilith's own timeframe, at the conclusion of this first instalment of the Xenogenesis trilogy, she is merely informed by Nikanj that she has already been impregnated. Thus, the threat of forced pregnancy that has hung over Lilith throughout the novel becomes a reality. However, what is important in the above excerpt is the evidence that the Oankali do not actually need biological pregnancy to achieve their crossbreeding goals. The reproductive horrors visited on the human survivors on the Oankali ship are thus strictly unnecessary.

The superfluity of human biological gestation for achieving the Oankali's objectives is more explicitly highlighted when Joseph confronts Nikanj about the proposed 'gene trade':

> 'You could clone us', Joseph said. 'Is that right?'
>
> 'Yes'.
>
> 'You could take reproductive cells from us and grow human embryos in artificial wombs?'
>
> 'Yes'.
>
> 'You can even re-create us from some kind of gene map or print'.
>
> 'We can do that too. We have already done these things. We must do them to understand a new species better. We must compare them to normal human conception and birth. We must compare the children we have made to those we took from Earth. We're very careful to avoid damaging new partner-species'.[121]

Herein lies the crux of the issue, the assumption that 'natural' gestation is necessarily better, and technological alternatives risk 'damaging' the offspring. Sanz Alonso also notes of this scene that:

> human beings become objects in the Oankali's hands; they are used as instruments without any value attached to human life itself. … Through instrumentalization the Oankali become the colonizers for whom human beings are just objects to experiment with, isolating and studying them.[122]

She notes the problem being dramatized here is not whether alien life exists and is coming to enslave humanity, but rather the ways human beings already instrumentalize each other and their environment, leading to destruction.[123] The 'gene trade' is presented in the text as inescapable, and thus, it is only the method of creating the hybrid children that could be the subject of potential negotiation. That the Oankali are unwilling to propose ectogenesis as a compromise that would greatly enhance the quality of life of the human survivors makes sense, given they seem to treat the species and their interests as inferior. However, the fact that Lilith never advocates for this, even after hearing Joseph's argument for it, is much more interesting. She too seems to suffer from a poverty of imagination regarding human reproductive futures.

Dawn is often classified as an Afrofuturist text, making it particularly noteworthy that post- and transhumanism are so violently opposed throughout. Sami Abdullah Al-Nuaimi et al. note that negativity regarding transhumanism is common in science fiction and is 'associated with the fear of human beings' annihilation and being othered as non-human beings'.[124] This is certainly a pervasive theme in *Dawn*. However, these authors claim Afrofuturism and transhumanism are typically 'linked together through utilising advanced technology for useful purposes and through the tendency for change'.[125] For

Florence Okoye, this change involves collectivist modes of technology use, rather than Western individualist accounts, suggesting 'Afrofuturism as intersectional transhumanism'.[126] However, this is definitely not how advanced technology is viewed in *Dawn*. Given Butler's reliance on sex-based genetic determinism in the text, it is possible to interpret the anti-technological elements of the story as not only highlighting a social resistance but also a supposed biological impossibility for change. As Jesser notes:

> Butler's essentialism should be read within a context of a gene theory that undermines racial categories and constructs, but that does abandon genetic input on other human aspects, most importantly, sex/gender. … Butler, while she undermines racial essentialism as corrupt and unscientific, retains a commitment to a qualified essentialist stance toward the biologically sexed body. [127]

The Oankali have described humans as fatally flawed because they possess 'a mismatched pair of genetic characteristics', namely, intelligence and hierarchical tendencies.[128] These are identified as candidates for correction via the ooloi's genetic engineering. Meanwhile, the physical and sexual violence perpetrated by human males is accepted as inevitable.[129] So too is a future where reproduction is still dependent on the exploitation of women's bodies, as even without the Oankali's interference, there is the assumption that the female survivors have a duty to procreate to save the species. This includes in their destined forest habitat, where pregnancy and childbirth are likely to entail significant loss of life due to lack of available medical care.

Dawn is clearly not proposing technology as a solution to sexual inequality in reproduction and its associated health risks; nevertheless, it contains a compelling argument for this conclusion. When considering the issue from within the fictional world Butler has created, what is preventing ectogenesis from being viewed as a serious alternative to biological gestation is the same thing that prevents Joseph's rape from being acknowledged as such: the point of view the narrative adopts.

Narratological analysis and point of view in *Dawn*

As discussed earlier, fiction has a role in fostering the 'moral emotions' and often achieves this through encouraging identification with and sympathy for specific characters.[130] In *Dawn*, Lilith is not only the protagonist, but the third-person narration is focalized through her. This is clear from the very opening of the novel:

> Alive!
> Still alive.
> Alive ... again.
>
> Awakening was hard, as always. The ultimate disappointment.
>
> ...
>
> At an earlier Awakening, she had decided that reality was whatever happened, whatever she perceived.[131]

Thus, the reader is informed upfront that what they are about to encounter is Lilith's perspective on the events of the narrative. This is important not only because of the limitations of awareness the previous discussion elucidated but also because Lilith has some unique views on human reproduction that may be influencing what the reader is able to access. While still living on Earth before the war, she had chosen to have a 'natural childbirth', without painkillers or hospital admission – 'Just something called a birthing center – a place for pregnant women who don't like the idea of being treated as though they were sick'.[132] Paul suggests this is why the Oankali selected her as their emissary, stating: 'You're probably just what they want in ways I haven't even thought of'.[133] It is unsurprising that a character who would denounce the over-medicalization of pregnancy and childbirth in general would be particularly opposed to more advanced interventions into human reproduction, including genetic engineering and artificial gestation. Osherow also notes that Lilith has the reader's sympathy partly due to her 'dire likeness' to Black women slaves from history, whose vulnerability to sexual assaults she claims is mirrored in Lilith's being violated throughout the text 'so thoroughly that human sex is no longer a possibility for her'.[134] Such a character provides a site for feminist resistance against gender-based oppression and colonial violence. She is also the very embodiment of the equity argument against emerging reproductive biotechnologies being released into the world without careful consideration of distributive justice demands, as well as protections for abortion rights.

While the focalization of *Dawn* may limit the explicit discussion of such matters, a bioethics-in-literature approach can open up this imaginative space. As mentioned in the previous chapter, working within the narrative logic of the story and its fictional world presents an opportunity to consider how the transhumanist interventions proposed in the novel *could* function in a way that avoids the dystopia. The overall conclusion of such an analysis would likely yield the answer: consent. Had the human survivors welcomed hybridization as a means of species survival, the central horror of the text would evaporate. However, the text is also able to illustrate how consent can be complicated by relative disadvantage, desperation and other situational elements. After all, despite being horrified by genetic engineering, Lilith 'consents' to various genetic adjustments to gain specific freedoms. Extrapolating to other reproductive biotechnologies reiterates the importance of considering how consent might be challenged by pronatalism, sexual inequality and other factors, without requiring the abandonment of a liberal approach that would support the rights of individuals to settle on their own definition of family and preferred methods of family creation.

This latter point introduces another consequence of adopting Lilith's point of view in the narrative: her implicit rejection of individual liberties in favour of collectivism. Hoda M. Zaki claims that 'the communitarian impulse borne of the merging of individuals with the group often figures as a desideratum in feminist utopian SF', but that in *Dawn*, this impulse is shown to be problematic as it depends on 'non-verbal communication ... as the means for resolving differences in points of view and thereby achieving unity'.[135] She notes that this is 'a human impossibility, given the nature of our language and how we use it'.[136] Lilith's self-serving representation of Joseph's rape as a source of enjoyment seems to support this argument. The reader is not invited into Joseph's inner world, so has nothing but his spoken dialogue to gain an insight into his perspective. This dialogue paints a very different picture to the narrator's account. But when it comes to appropriating the voice of others, Zaki claims Butler's novels 'contain an implicit and internal critique of and rebuke to one aspect of liberal feminist ideology: its claim to speak for all women, regardless of color or class'.[137] Ironically, this is exactly what Lilith seems to do throughout her mothering mission – it is not just that she wants all the human survivors to believe the same thing and act in the same way, she specifically needs them to accept her version of reality and work towards her vision of future community.

Another important narratological technique exposed in the quote at the opening of this section is the use of free indirect discourse (FID).[138] In her article on narrative voice, Julie Choi describes FID as 'the effect created by the translation of what "sounds" like first-person or direct discourse, in the present of "speech" or "thought", into the third-person past of the narrative'.[139] Unlike in external narration, such as the introduction 'Lilith Iyapo lay gasping, shaking with the force of her effort',[140] in which the perspective provided comes from outside, FID is described by Gertrude Schuelke as a 'slipping' into the character's own words, for the purpose of providing an insight into that character's personal perspective or consciousness.[141] FID typically lacks qualifiers such as 'he said' or 'she thought' in the narrative, making it harder to separate from an omniscient external narrator. In his article, 'Dual Perspective', Paul Hernadi refers to this as a 'lack of *verbum dicendi*', leading to FID assuming the 'grammatical disguise of narrated fact'.[142] In other words, because it is unclear to the reader that a character is 'speaking', it can look as if the information conveyed is objective truth, rather than just one person's perspective. But while FID may present the illusion of direct communication between the character and the reader, the narrator is still mediating the exchange.

While there is some disagreement among narratologists regarding what constitutes FID, there is still a general consensus that there must be a smooth transition between the external third-person (heterodiegetic) narrator and the assumed voice of the character, as demonstrated by the continued use of past tense and third-person pronouns. In the case of the opening lines of *Dawn*, this refers to the continued use of Lilith's 'she', despite clearly communicating things that are not narrated facts, but rather the character's personal opinions. Being awake is not *objectively* the 'ultimate disappointment', it is merely Lilith's present context that makes it so for *her*. Another example of FID can be seen in the following excerpt:

> There had been healing in the long sleep. She Awoke with no particular inclination to speak her thoughts aloud or cry or sit on the floor and rock backward and forward, but her memory was unimpaired. She remembered all too well the long period of silence and isolation. Even an unseen inquisitor was preferable.[143]

In the above example, FID occurs when the reader can sense the impartiality of the external narrator being dissolved and replaced with Lilith's personal perspective. The judgement that any company is better than total isolation is one that may not be universally shared among the captives, and yet it is presented as fact. Dorrit Cohn refers to such a technique as a 'superimposing' of the character's voice onto the narrator's, allowing the narrator to articulate feelings and attitudes of the character not otherwise manifest in their behaviour or quoted speech.[144] Thus, FID can be said to expose the narrator's appropriation of the character's voice while attempting to explore what is going on in that character's mind. Importantly, the use of FID here introduces the possibility of unreliability – if the reader cannot trust that 'an unseen inquisitor' is, in fact, 'preferable' to no company at all, they might also question the earlier narrated claims that Lilith has fully recovered from her mental breakdown or retained her full memory of past events.

According to Yael Sharvit, the use of the 'temporal perspective' of the character is a necessary requirement for FID, always referring to the character's 'now'.[145] In *Dawn*, the only histories and explanations the reader gains access to are the ones from Lilith's perspective, for example, describing her own past experiences of pregnancy, or those provided to her through direct dialogue with another character. By extension, Lilith can easily reject ectogenesis because to her, pregnancy and childbirth are achievable (and survivable) without any medical or technological intervention: 'It wasn't any fun, but it went ok', she says.[146] As with many of the other science-fictional texts considered in this book, it would be interesting to consider the value of reproductive biotechnologies from the perspective of a character struggling with fertility or unable to gestate.

Another element of FID exposed in the above passage is the exploitation of the 'stylistic peculiarities' of the character's speech.[147] The word 'inquisitor' sounds like it has come from Lilith's vocabulary, as a student of cultural history, and represents her own linguistic biases. Stefan Oltean notes that the language of FID commonly employs the 'idiosyncratic lexical elements' of the assumed character's speech, including the use of slang and colloquialisms as used by the character in direct dialogue or internal monologue.[148] There are relatively few examples of internal monologue provided in the text, but these tend to occur when Lilith is in conversation with one of the Oankali and consciously not saying what she is thinking. In these cases, the narrative retains the marker 'she thought', clearly distinguishing thought from speech. The use of a character's distinctive speech pattern in FID allows the reader to interpret the narrative in light of their knowledge of the character involved to determine whether the narration is likely to be reliable. This is of particular interest when deciding whether a specific description is intended literally or metaphorically and whether it is realistic or likely to be exaggerated. As such, it becomes clear that interfering with 'natural' human reproduction is a source of horror in *Dawn*, because it is horrific *to Lilith*. The reader does not receive this message with this qualifier though; through internal focalization and FID, they receive it as fact.

There are limited examples of FID in *Dawn* that are not adopting Lilith's perspective, but their rarity makes them all the more significant. One example can be seen following the death of one of the more violent human men, Peter, after he realizes he has been drugged and sexually exploited by his assigned ooloi:

> he apparently decided he had been humiliated and enslaved. The drug seemed to him to be not a less painful way of getting used to frightening non-humans, but a way of turning him against himself, causing him to demean himself in alien perversions. His humanity was profaned. His manhood was taken away.[149]

The 'apparently' seems to be Lilith's voice, whereas the final two sentences are (arguably) Peter's. No mimetic speech from Peter's perspective on the matter is provided, so this 'slipping' into his character's perspective is the only insight the reader gains into his mental state at the time he attacks and is accidentally killed by the ooloi. This is different to how another character's violent outburst is handled in the text, with his friend describing their understanding of his motivations in direct speech:

> 'Look at things from Curt's point of view', Gabriel said. 'He's not in control even of what his own body does and feels. He's taken like a woman … He can't let them get away with that'.[150]

Although the content is similar, the different narrative techniques produce a very different effect on how this content is communicated. In the second example, it is clear the reader is hearing a specific character's interpretation of events, and it is thus open for debate, while in the first, the narrative perspective is presented as truth.

As has been demonstrated throughout this chapter, employing literary and narratological tools of analysis to science-fictional representations of reproductive futures can help articulate complex bioethical issues, such as the challenge of obtaining informed consent under conditions of uncertainty or systemic disadvantage. It also helps consider how narrative framing and voice can manipulate how new technologies are positioned and represented, by only telling part of the story or only considering some points of view. As a final consideration, this chapter will now consider how science fiction can contribute to the practical design of emerging reproductive technologies and their future regulation, drawing on *Dawn* and several other works considered in earlier chapters.

Design ethics for the artificial womb

Design ethics refers to the incorporation of ethical values and principles into product design. Peter-Paul Verbeek states that for emerging technologies, this involves being conscious of the social impact such technologies will have as soon as they are released into society.[151] For ectogenesis, this requires an awareness of the potential threats to equity and abortion rights discussed in earlier chapters, so the design and release of the technology can be done in such a way as to mitigate these threats. Design ethics also requires an appreciation of how imagery impacts ethical judgement regarding reproductive biotechnologies, such that the visual appearance of the artificial womb can avoid triggering feelings of disgust or discomfort in prospective parents. This is precisely where 'visual bioethics' might help tease out the ramifications of product design decisions in reproductive medicine, facilitating a design ethics approach. Using the related term 'value sensitive design' and applying it specifically to the development of the artificial placenta, Romanis et al. advocate for design choices that focus on 'efficacy, compassion and accessibility' and consider how various options might impact the interactions between prospective parents and their developing offspring.[152] Romanis and Victoria Adkins add to this discussion that the protocols for partial ectogenesis also need to be 'loss-sensitive', given that many women faced with the need for such interventions will have recently experienced an interruption to a biological pregnancy they may not have wanted or foreseen.[153]

Visual aspects of artificial womb design are important, as research indicates parents of premature infants often struggle to cope with the confronting image of their under-developed newborn, reliant on medical technologies, and that the separation while their child is in the NICU can affect bonding.[154] For offspring being gestated in an artificial womb, the same potentially distressing elements will be present, but over an even longer time period.[155] While some prospective parents may value the opportunity to observe a greater scope of foetal development, others may find this disconcerting. Again, using the example of the NICU, some parents report feeling obligated to spend as much time with their infant as possible, a sense of never being 'off duty'[156] that it would be impractical to replicate in the artificial gestation scenario. A design ethics approach would consider how the artificial womb should look, who should have access to view the developing foetus within and whether there are grounds to limit exposure to these images to prevent psychological distress.[157] From a logistical perspective, it would also consider the best materials and appearance to promote healthy foetal development, for example, whether lighting and colour schemes should be designed to imitate the levels and shades found in the organic womb.

In Butler's *Dawn*, the artificial wombs used in the Oankali's human experiments are never described; however, extrapolating from the rest of their technology, it can be assumed the system would have demonstrated a similar intersection of organic and synthetic components as their ship. Several critics also refer to the process of Awakening the other humans as a form of childbirth, describing the individual suspended animation enclosures as 'wombs'.[158] Indeed, as Lilith liberates each new member from the modified carnivorous plants, the scenes are reminiscent of the births shown in the film *The Island*, as described in Chapter 2.

Considering the aesthetics of some of the other representations of ectogenesis in science fiction discussed in earlier chapters also demonstrates how fictional imagery can contribute to design ethics and the conceptualization of speculative technologies. By recognizing the impact of the 'yuck factor' in ethical judgement, the physical object of the artificial womb can be designed in a way that avoids such negative connotations. In other words, the horrific and repulsive images of ectogenesis seen in *The Matrix* and *The Island*, for example, provide a map for what *not* to do. In Chapter 1, it was also noted that various commentators and scientists were unable to visualize full ectogenesis because they were extrapolating from existing technologies, rather than considering a more integrated organic-synthetic interaction. The imagination of a science fiction author is not impeded thus.

Immega's visual description of the prototype artificial womb used in *Super-Earth Mother* (2023) is a good example of the scientific imaginary manifesting in science fiction. Expanding the quote provided in Chapter 3 yields the fuller context:

> 'I've reviewed your artificial womb design', he announced. 'It looks simple – a bag of seawater in a box with some pumps and filters'.
>
> The man knew nothing. 'Those are just 'bio-bags'' for a fetus removed from the natural mother. My womb does full ectogenesis. It can grow an embryo from a fertilized egg and bring the fetus to term'.
>
> Kelso raised his bushy eyebrows. 'How does it do that?'
>
> 'I designed an artificial uterus that supplies blood to a natural placenta. It uses a semipermeable membrane that's connected to a miniature heart-lung machine'.[159]

Earlier, this same technician (Jenica) is seen monitoring her ectogenesis experiment, leading to a description of the foetus involved as well:

> She turned to a lab bench and adjusted a pump connected to a stainless oven with a transparent dome top. A large display showed ever-changing graphs that wiggled across the screen. Then it cycled to show an ultrasound display of a

> fetus that looked several months old. It twisted, kicking its legs, and sucked its thumb.[160]

This description is normalizing and even cute. However, when further described as being the result of 'no eggs, no sperm, no impregnation – immaculate conception', the foetus is immediately re-cast in the internal monologue of the witness as 'transhuman', with Kelso asking himself if its existence is even legal.[161] Nevertheless, the vision of ectogenesis here is scientifically compelling, with the integration of an organic placenta suggesting one way the technical gaps in artificial gestation could be approached. The significance of terminology is also addressed when Jenica explains her '*bea-u-tiful boy*' will be 'hatched' from his 'metallic egg' in a few months.[162] This also explains that the foetus being viewed in the earlier quote is already quite well developed. To consider the potential psychological impact of being able to witness even earlier stages of development, *The Pod Generation* (2023) provides a more useful example.

The translucent, egg-shaped pods in *The Pod Generation* bear some similarity to the description in Immega's text, also boasting an app-linked 'thriving chart' that parents can use to continually monitor their foetus. In addition, during the tour of the Womb Center facility, prospective parents are shown the fingerprint scanner that can be used to open a viewing panel in the pod, with everyone cooing when they see a foetus floating peacefully within. While Alvy is initially repulsed by the artificial pod, complaining it is made from 'plastic … chemicals and petroleum derivatives and silicone', he eventually grows attached to it, as described in Chapter 3.[163] However, the film also shows his discomfort when the moment of conception is taken from the private, sexual space and magnified on a screen in the medical clinic room. As the director narrates the process almost like a sports commentator, it has an emasculating effect for Alvy whose sperm are the subject of the race. After the process, the couple are left in a room with their zygote in a cannister, their nurse implying this is a significant milestone, while they just look confused and underwhelmed. A comparison can be drawn with how bringing sonogram pictures home has become a cultural milestone of pregnancy, except with the perpetual visibility of a foetus in an artificial womb meaning there may be no limit to the number of developmental events that can be marked. The Womb Center staff seem at least partially aware of the potential downsides of this, as they strictly limit the time parents can have their pod at home with them.

The Pod Generation also explores what male pregnancy – albeit artificial – may look like, although this is mostly viewed through the female gaze and often negatively. Men are humorously seen blundering around with the egg-shaped pods strapped to them, with Alvy's preference for wearing his on the front seen to be 'reckless'. Nevertheless, it is the ability for him to experience even this small imitation of gestation that ultimately leaves his partner feeling like she is one failing to bond with the foetus by comparison. When Rachel decides to wear the pod herself to work to redress this, she accidentally walks it into a glass door and is later advised to plug the pod into a closet charging station rather than have it at her desk, making her look like 'the distracted mom'. Although she initially tried to fit the pod under her jumper, mimicking a physically pregnant body, even when in full view, Rachel misjudges her new physical dimensions and struggles to adapt. Importantly, her awkwardness is exaggerated as she relates feeling disconnected from her offspring precisely because she has opted out of an embodied pregnancy. The fact that she can choose which days to be inconvenienced by the additional weight of her pod sets her apart from the physically pregnant characters she interacts with, who move gracefully despite their bigger sizes.

In her article, 'Visibly Pregnant', JaneMaree Maher notes that pregnant women's bodies naturally occupy 'new spatial co-ordinates' over the gestational period while remaining 'a still-unified corporeal space'.[164] She notes that when fiction tries to replicate this for male protagonists, it brings attention to how the changes in women's bodies during pregnancy are often accepted uncritically. Using the example of *Junior* (1994), where Arnold Schwarzenegger's character, Dr Alex Hesse, volunteers to be the first pregnant man, Maher states:

> *Junior* makes clear that, since women seemingly enter this embodied state without thinking, they cannot achieve the transformative benefits that accrue to men. Male pregnancy requires attachment by intention and control: scientific, emotional and visual. Men can choose a relationship with pregnancy; one that extends and improves them. Women are always already almost pregnant; actually becoming so doesn't change them.[165]

Alvy chooses to undergo this same transformation without the need for the physicality of pregnancy, whereas Rachel is seen to lose something valuable when challenging the assumption that her body should change to facilitate family making. She even suggests that the time Alvy spent with the pod meant he got 'the hormones', making him more ready for parenthood than she is. From a design ethics perspective, considering how bonding may be enhanced for all prospective parents through promoting interactions with the developing foetus may necessitate similar considerations as are seen in *The Pod Generation*, when characters discuss the battery life of the pods and how long they can safely be removed from the Womb Center facility. Whether an artificial womb should be designed to be portable or fixed, visible or shielded, an imitation of the organic womb or unapologetically synthetic, are all relevant questions science-fictional representations can help explore.

To explore the impact of artistic representations of ectogenesis on public opinion, the team at Eindhoven who are creating the first prototype artificial womb, engaged with designers during Dutch Design Week in 2018, leading to the speculative design exhibition, *Reprodutopia*.[166] This exhibition contained an artist's impression of the artificial womb that Patricia De Vries described as resembling a 'bunch of air-filled, flesh-colored balls look[ing] eerily like loitering testicles'.[167] Despite this 'tragicomic' outcome, she claims:

> Artistic representations of reproductive technologies – be it in film, literature, or speculative art practices – can show us how people relate to these technologies. Art practices contribute to the materialization of shared norms and values.[168]
>
> ...
>
> What speculative art and design add to the sciences are tools and resources to reflect on social norms and values, anxieties, expectations, and desires braided around emerging technologies.[169]

Specifically mentioning Butler's *Dawn* as an example of such an imagining, she notes: 'Stories we *do* tell about the future of reproduction – whether imagined in the form of design-fiction, narrativized in science-fiction, or represented in films – are situated and embedded', including through specific cultural histories.[170] In other words, these fictional representations have come from somewhere, they are powerful, and they are not neutral. Joyce Nabuurs et al.'s study of the visualizations of potential artificial womb designs shown in *Reprodutopia* sought to answer the question of 'whether speculative design can facilitate pragmatist reflective inquiry; activating publics to perform a dramatic rehearsal and use their moral imagination to make sense of the soft impacts of emerging science and technology'.[171] This study confirmed a role for the imagination in helping integrate novel technologies into society and facilitating public understanding, with various respondents also discussing how the appearance of the artificial womb models impacted their response to the technology. These insights could influence both the practical and ethical design choices made by scientists working in this area, aiming to develop a user-centred design. As such, it is worth considering how such images and imaginings can be incorporated into a theory of anticipatory, or speculative bioethics.

Anticipatory ethics for emerging technologies

Combining the above elements illustrates how science fiction can contribute to an overarching anticipatory ethics for emerging technologies, including ectogenesis, which considers different points of view regarding the appropriate design, implementation and evaluation of new reproductive futures. Much like the science fiction genre, anticipatory ethics has various names and definitions, but most involve some use of speculation to predict, forewarn and potentially mitigate ethical issues arising in emerging technologies. Using the term 'speculative bioethics', Tess Johnson and Elizabeth Chloe Romanis provide a useful review of possible methodologies, stating these:

> include a range of forms of inquiry, all related by being – at their core – a form of practical/applied ethics in relation to less temporally immediate problems from a range of contextual possibilities not limited to, but including, imaginaries, thought experiments, and future technologies.[172]

These authors note '[s]peculation affords researchers room for imagination', creating a space for 'novel thinking and argumentation'.[173] This is reminiscent of Le Guin's claims about science fiction providing a safe space for social and scientific experimentation.[174] As the genre that speculates on socio-technical futures, science fiction is particularly well suited to inform anticipatory ethics and governance. Thought experimentation is useful precisely because it demands an interrogation of the contextual assumptions that might otherwise be taken for granted, with science fiction narratives imagining entire worlds where these assumptions may be rewritten. And as Johnson and Romanis note, the value of speculative discussions of emerging technologies is not limited to 'what we ought to do *in the advent of the technology*', because many of the ethical issues identified – for example, inequalities, distributive justice issues, etc. – already exist in the present and are merely magnified by considering the addition of a novel technology.[175] As such, even if human ectogenesis is never fully realized, the ethical issues identified in science-fictional representations of this technology are still worth debating. Johnson and Romanis conclude:

> Speculative work can be important in raising public awareness and excitement about novel technologies, or even about the field of bioethics in general. It can be important in informing policymaking in matters only slightly related to the actual speculative work. What's more, speculation is crucial in preparing the field and the public for involvement in translational discussions of emerging technologies in the future. The law and public policy are always struggling to

> keep up with scientific development (often because other matters are considered more urgent until the development itself becomes the urgent matter). One of the great advantages of bioethics is that we have the luxury of not falling into this same trap.[176]

As noted in the previous chapter, the qualities that can classify a work as science fiction also make a text adept at this future speculation. However, when considering the radical potential of utopian narratives to influence social structures, Latimer brings attention to the fact that most supposedly disruptive reproductive technologies in the past have simply been subsumed into existing institutions and power structures.[177] She cites as evidence Franklin's claims about the 'everydayness of IVF',[178] a technology Mason relates was initially met with anxiety due to concerns the children born using the technique would not be 'wholly human'.[179] Once these fears were shown to be unfounded, the technology was simply incorporated into business as usual. Far from undermining heteronormative family structures, initial access protocols for IVF rather reinforced these, including by restricting access for socially infertile individuals and couples. At least at the outset, the release of the technology failed to achieve its utopian potential of equalizing reproduction for same-sex couples.

Eric Racine et al. provide a useful account of anticipatory ethics in their article on cognitive enhancement, noting that critics of the practice are concerned that bioethical analyses grounded in 'highly speculative claims may reflect and encourage technological determinism', while also engaging in slippery slope argumentation and 'conjuring up hyperbolic or unreasonable scenarios', including ones that might lead to unrealistic expectations of new technologies among consumers.[180] These authors claim such use of speculation in bioethics can lead to 'a misalignment between the reality of scientific and clinical evidence and bioethical discussion [that] negatively impacts the credibility of bioethics', while also focusing attention on more sensational media accounts of emerging technologies and therapies in a way that may distract from more immediate bioethical issues.[181] However, on the positive side, they welcome the role of speculation in enabling 'the foresight of ethical problems before a novel technology is introduced or disseminated' and suggest that practical methods of health technology assessment may pursue similar goals, allowing proactive ethical assessment of the impact of future technologies on society.[182]

Extrapolating to fictional worlds where ectogenesis has already been implemented, considering the socio-political structures in these alternate societies may allow for more equitable distribution systems to be designed in advance of the technology in the real world. This could aim at avoiding repetition or exacerbation of existing inequalities of access and outcome through speculation and anticipation of the likely consequences of this technology on concepts of family. As such, exploring science fiction narratives, including through the tools of literary analysis and narratology outlined above, may elucidate relevant ethical principles or enhance moral intuitions that can inform ethical guidelines and policies for research and development. This further explains why the shift to a narrative focus when considering the artificial womb is an ethical shift, as it capitalizes on the contribution of moral emotions, spectatorship and visual bioethics on the development and implementation of this emerging technology with significant potential to alter social structures and human relationships.

When it comes to the predictable threat to abortion rights that ectogenesis might entail in some jurisdictions, science fiction also provides useful data. As Sarah Langford notes:

> Ectogenesis will never end the need for abortion, because abortion arises from gendered social conditions that place women at risk of unwanted pregnancy. Radical feminists understand that the only 'solution' to abortion is to ensure women's freedom from rape and from compulsory heterosexuality, and their access to completely safe and effective contraception.[183]

When a utopian narrative has incorporated ectogenesis but failed to achieve sexual equality, these other social concerns might provide an explanation. For example, the technology in *The Pod Generation* may have removed the need for career women to be pregnant, but it has not improved maternal health for the socio-economically disadvantaged nor challenged managerial assumptions about female employees being less committed to their jobs once they become mothers. There is also no mention of how unwanted biological pregnancies are handled in this fictional world. Meanwhile, a tale like *The Left Hand of Darkness* can achieve the same goal Farquhar claims for reproductive technologies in general, namely, to 'change and challenge the fetishizing of blood ties, the nuclear romance of reproduction, and their concomitant sexual desires'.[184] It does this by exploring the suite of social changes required to promote equality in reproduction, rather than a single intervention.

Science fiction stories, even including purely dystopian visions of the future, can help anticipate what other changes would need to attend the advent of ectogenesis technology in the real world to support the technology in enhancing reproductive options for some without causing harm to others. However, as Belling notes:

> Close attention to authorial agenda, rhetorical effect, cultural context, and reader response is needed to understand the unruly contribution of these texts to bioethics discourse. Fiction is a way of knowing that can be modulated but never determined by an author's earnest framing or a publisher's sensationalist marketing. Yet it can certainly influence decisions and policy-making.[185]

Thus, it is important to interrogate the choice and use of science-fictional stories in bioethics, as the different perspectives included might help pre-empt group-specific concerns about emerging technologies, as demonstrated in the Butler case study. At the same time, both the cautionary aspect of many science-fictional narratives and the detailed characters and fictional world-building provide valuable content for anticipatory ethics, expanding imaginative possibilities and moral spectatorship.

Conclusion

In conclusion, the development of ectogenesis could confer significant benefits on many women and play a vital role in promoting sexual equality in human reproduction. However, it would also require a reimagining of the legal and moral status of the embryo, the cultural significance of pregnancy and childbirth and the dominant perceptions of gender roles in procreation. At present, outdated laws based on doomsday predictions of potential future misuse of emerging reproductive technologies hamper research into this equalizing alternative to physical gestation. Science fiction provides a safe space to test out ethical theories regarding ectogenesis, presenting fictional worlds in which this technology already exists and exploring how this has impacted society. While there are positive representations of the technology in the genre, for the most part, ectogenesis is depicted negatively in science fiction. Furthermore, when science-fictional references appear in bioethics scholarship focused on reproductive technologies, the choice of texts is almost exclusively dystopian. Science fiction stories, and particularly utopian and dystopian narratives, are persuasive agents for social change; however, this selective use of the genre only promotes a techno-conservative agenda. The power of science fiction in bioethics indicates there may be an ethical obligation to avoid simply exploiting the overly negative representations of ectogenesis found within the genre and, instead, engage in close textual analysis of the themes and motifs present in the text. Given the necessity of thinking beyond the confines of current legal and medical practice in bioethical debate, a poverty of imagination regarding potentially equalizing alternatives to biological gestation limits the scope of discussion.

Feminist utopias are particularly valuable to any discussion of 'bioethics-in-literature', as they explore what changes may be necessary in the present in order to confront sexual inequality and promote a more equitable future.[1] Rudy notes that utopias like Piercy's *Woman on the Edge of Time* and Le Guin's *The Left*

Hand of Darkness expose audiences to an estranged reality in which 'women's bodies are not the only places babies can grow'.[2] Such a radical shift challenges assumptions about gender roles and secures the position of science fiction as a site to consider possible futures and the cultural meaning of reproduction and motherhood.[3] Ruth Levitas notes that while dystopian fiction 'can be a vehicle of resistance, it is much less able to register transformation and redemption. It may point to the exit, but it does not suggest what we might find, or make, when we leave.'[4] When considering the goal of achieving sexual equality in human reproduction, feminist utopias can provide a map to follow. Further engagement with these texts in bioethics scholarship could help balance the debate regarding the desirability of ectogenesis and other reproductive technologies.

Future research directions

Cannold claims that severance theorists[5] and those adhering to a 'right to life' anti-abortion stance are logically committed to support ectogenesis as an alternative to unwanted pregnancy that does not lead to the termination of foetal life.[6] However, the qualitative studies she published in the early to mid-90s indicated women's attitudes towards ectogenesis did not line up with this notion. Segers reminds us that in interpreting Cannold's results 'caution is in order due to the small, unrepresentative sample, the risks of making anachronous extrapolations, and the difficulty of full appeal to empirical findings in assessing emerging technology'.[7] Nevertheless, future research could aim to compare attitudes today to those in Cannold's pioneering study, especially in the light of recent legal challenges to abortion rights, including since the overturning of *Roe v Wade* in the United States.

A major gap in the current scholarship on ectogenesis ethics that also needs to be urgently addressed is the potential role of this emerging technology in less affluent contexts or where there is significant wealth disparity. While the unequal distribution of maternal health risks across populations, both within and across countries, is well documented, how the release of ectogenesis technologies could impact this *globally* is rarely considered seriously. Gabriela Arguedas-Ramírez and Danielle M. Wenner support the development of a global feminist ethics for dealing with reproductive technology, particularly in a post-*Roe* world where various countries are rolling back women's reproductive rights.[8] Similarly, Gisela Zaremberg et al. claim that feminist discourse in parts of Latin America has shifted away from fighting for more rights to defending existing rights from being taken away, saying this 'echoes the experiences of feminists around the world who find themselves defending women's rights – if not their and their communities' very lives – in hostile times, devoting much of their energy to preserving previous achievements'.[9] As with all areas of healthcare resource allocation, decisions regarding who will have access to emerging reproductive technologies, for what purposes and who will pay will be politically and culturally motivated.

Further exploring the political implications of ectogenesis, in her article, 'Gestation, Equality and Freedom: Ectogenesis as a Political Perspective', Giulia Cavaliere writes:

> Ectogenesis is considered to be equality-promoting on two accounts: it promotes equality between men and women, and between biologically and socially infertile and fertile women. Despite this depiction, the reach of defences of ectogenesis appears limited. While health-related risks, burdens and deaths caused by gestation and childbirth affect all women and can indeed be framed in terms of a 'natural inequality', they are not equally distributed among all women. Documented evidence shows that women belonging to ethnic minorities, poor and disabled women are at a much higher risk of experiencing complications during gestation and childbirth and of dying as a result of these complications.
>
> Now, one could argue that for ectogenesis to be equality-promoting, these groups may just need to be prioritised in their access to this practice (or at least their access to this practice would have to be secured). This would at least represent an incremental improvement of the status quo. There are, however, two sorts of barriers to achieving this: financial and cultural. Concerning financial barriers, Kendal's central claim in her defence of ectogenesis is that this practice should be state-sponsored to promote and secure equal opportunities for women. Similarly, Smajdor argues that natural inequalities 'may generate a prima facie right to restitution'. However, while I agree with Smajdor and Kendal on normative aspects of their proposals, I am sceptical as to their feasibility.[10]

These feasibility concerns must be addressed for ectogenesis to reach its potential as an equalizing technology. Again, we have lessons to learn from both the history of reproductive biotechnology development and the realm of science fiction. Similar accusations of inequitable distribution were levelled at IVF when it was first released, and it is certainly still the case that even those countries providing state sponsorship have not achieved equality either in access or outcomes across populations of women.[11] Likewise, fictional narratives where reproductive technologies are widely (or even universally) distributed still often depict significant social inequality. However, the argument that state-level financial constraints inevitably condemn ectogenesis to exacerbating existing inequalities in healthcare fails to recognize that large enough resources to support universal (maternal) healthcare do exist in many jurisdictions; they are simply being directed elsewhere. Governments may currently be more motivated to subsidize fossil fuel companies, invest in specific military projects or provide tax cuts to the wealthy, but this does not mean such priorities should be considered insurmountable or eternal. As with many resource allocation dilemmas, particularly in Western bioethical debate, conditions of scarcity in public healthcare systems have often been artificially created.[12] Romanis also reminds us that there is currently a lack of empirical evidence on how reproductive rights organizations and political advocates perceive the equality-enhancing potential of ectogenesis.[13]

Another future research direction that could be pursued regarding the role of science fiction in bioethical debate might include further empirical studies on the impact of reading certain types of stories on short- and long-term attitudes towards marginalized groups and emerging technologies. A more thorough understanding of how fiction evokes empathy for others and how this might be used positively could yield significant social benefits. Alexandra Krendel and Mike Ryder's 2025 article, 'Role of Science Fiction in Conceptualising the Reproductive Future', already highlights what they refer to as a 'critical gap' in discussions of full ectogenesis that ignore science fiction's influence, 'as fiction is central to how the public make sense of new technologies'.[14] Achieving a more nuanced approach to the use of science fiction in bioethics scholarship that demonstrates greater respect for textual fidelity and the tools of literary analysis would be a valuable goal in this future research endeavour. The immediate next step for this project though is to codify a 'creative utopian bioethics methodology' that is replicable, teachable and applicable not only to the analysis of bioethically informed science fiction utopian narratives, as is seen here, but also to their creation.

Overall, this book has argued that science fiction has the potential to contribute meaningfully to the imaginative work of bioethics. The representation of ectogenesis and other reproductive technologies provides a good case study for exploring what changes need to take place for this potential to be realized in the future. Such change is likely to happen only by degrees and may never fully reach its potential. Nevertheless, striving toward a 'utopian' goal for the relationship between the narrative genres of science fiction and bioethics is a worthwhile endeavour, particularly given the potential for this relationship to challenge existing assumptions about human reproduction. To adapt Suvin's definition of utopia, the use of science-fictional texts and images need not be *perfectly* deployed in bioethics – merely *more perfectly* than the current reductive modes seen in scholarship. This book has explored a selection of methods that could be used to achieve this end, promoting the idea that an ethical encounter with narrative art involves allowing texts to challenge and instruct – to use us, rather than be used by us, to explore alternatives to the real world.

Notes

Introduction

1 Megan-Jane Johnstone, 'Ethics and Ectogenesis', *Australian Nursing Journal* 33, no. 11 (2010): 33.

2 There is some disagreement in the literature regarding the correct term here, with ectogestation, artificial womb technology, *ex vivo* gestation and *ex utero* gestation all used by different authors. For consistency, this book will predominantly use ectogenesis, and, unless otherwise stated, this will refer to full ectogenesis, e.g., gestation in an artificial womb from conception to 'birth'.

3 As far as is logically consistent, throughout this text, the term 'woman' should be read as inclusively as possible, referring to cis- and transgender women and to those who are physiologically and socially fertile or infertile. As some discussions are focused on biological reproductive capabilities, where a more 'nuts and bolts' approach to sexual difference is relevant, this should be clear from context. It is recognized that some of the discussions regarding pregnant people will only be applicable to physiologically fertile cisgender women and some transgender men and non-binary individuals, so this is sometimes specifically noted for clarity. It is also important to note that biological differences are dynamic, and as sexual and reproductive medicine continue to advance, these distinctions are likely to change.

4 Jennifer S. Hendricks, 'Not of Woman Born: A Scientific Fantasy', *Case Western Reserve Law Review* 62 (2012): 10.

5 Anna Smajdor, 'The Moral Imperative for Ectogenesis', *Cambridge Quarterly Healthcare Ethics* 16, no. 3 (2007): 340; World Health Organization, 'Managing Complications in Pregnancy and Childbirth: A Guide for Midwives and Doctors – Second Edition', February 2017. Accessed 29 January 2025. https://www.who.int/publications/i/item/9789241565493

6 Sophie Lewis, *Full Surrogacy Now: Feminism Against Family* (London: Verso Books, 2019), 1. Here, Lewis also notes: 'The everyday "miracle" that transpires in pregnancy, the production of that number more than one and less than two, receives more idealizing lip-service than it does respect', which is particularly relevant for future discussions of pronatalism.

7 Michael Olausson, et al., 'Ethics of Uterus Transplantation with Live Donors', *Fertility and Sterility* 102, no. 1 (2014): 40.

8 Giuliano Testa, et al., 'Uterus Transplant in Women with Absolute Uterine-Factor Infertility', *JAMA* 332, no. 10 (2024): 817–24.

9 Laura O'Donovan, Nicola Jane Williams and Stephen Wilkinson, 'Ethical and Policy Issues Raised by Uterus Transplants', *British Medical Bulletin* 131, no. 1 (2019): 19–28.

10 Evie Kendal and Julian J. Koplin, 'The Moral Superiority of Bioengineered Wombs and Ectogenesis for Absolute Uterine Factor Infertility', *Cambridge Quarterly of Healthcare Ethics* 31, no. 1 (2022): 73–82.

11 Yashita Khulbe, et al., 'Artificial Womb: Opportunities and Challenges for Public Health', *International Journal of Surgery* 109, no. 3 (2023): 618–19.

12 Zhelan Huang, Tiantian Xiao and Wenhao Zhou, 'Artificial Womb: A Paradigm Shift for Saving Extremely Premature Infants', *Chinese Medical Journal* 136, no. 14 (2023): 1759–61.

13 Frida Simonstein and Michal Mashiach-Eizenberg, 'The Artificial Womb: A Pilot Study Considering People's Views on the Artificial Womb and Ectogenesis in Israel', *Cambridge Quarterly of Healthcare Ethics* 18 (2009): 88.

14 Anna Smajdor, 'In Defense of Ectogenesis', *Cambridge Quarterly of Healthcare Ethics* 21, no. 1 (2012): 91.

15 This term is often used to mean an inability to even consider things beyond a narrow scope. In his book, *A Poverty of Imagination: Bootstrap Capitalism, Sequel to Welfare Reform* (Wisconsin: Wisconsin University Press, 2000), David Stoesz famously uses the term to capture the limited conception of welfare as a mere absence of material deprivation without any true reforms to tackle systemic poverty.

16 Diana Meyers, 'The Rush to Motherhood: Pronatalist Discourse and Women's Autonomy', *Signs* 26, no. 3 (2001): 752.

17 Ibid., 746.

18 In the future, alternative methods of gametogenesis may serve to remove the additional burden of oocyte retrieval for prospective parents and donors.

19 Rosemarie Tong, *Feminist Thought: A Comprehensive Introduction* (Boulder, Colorado: Westview Press, 1989), 75.

20 Ibid.

21 Evie Kendal, *Equal Opportunity and the Case for State Sponsored Ectogenesis* (Basingstoke: Palgrave Macmillan, 2015). This is the first major text of a body of work in this area published over the past ten years, with some other examples also listed in the bibliography for reference.

22 Dion Farquhar, *The Other Machine: Discourse and Reproductive Technologies* (New York: Routledge, 1996), 29.

23 Dennis Livingston, 'The Biology of Utopia: Science Fiction Perspectives on Ectogenesis', in *The Custom-made Child? Women-Centred Perspectives*, Helen B. Holmes, et al. (eds) (New Jersey: Humana Press, 1981), 281.

24 Eileen Gunn, 'How America's Leading Science Fiction Authors Are Shaping Your Future', *Smithsonian* Magazine, May 2014. Accessed 22 January 2024. https://www.smithsonianmag.com/arts-culture/how-americas-leading-science-fiction-authors-are-shaping-your-future-180951169/

25 Amy Mullin, 'Moral Defects, Aesthetic Defects, and the Imagination', *Journal of Aesthetics and Art Criticism* 62, no. 3 (2004): 249

26 Ibid., 250.

27 Ibid., 251.

28 Nobuya Unno, et al., 'Development of an Artificial Placenta: Survival of Isolated Goat Fetuses for Three Weeks with Umbilical Arteriovenous Extracorporeal Membrane Oxygenation', *Artificial Organs* 17, no. 12 (1993): 996–1003.

29 Shulamith Firestone, *The Dialectic of Sex: The Case for Feminist Revolution* (New York: William Morrow and Company, 1970).

30 Julien Murphy, 'Is Pregnancy Necessary? Feminist Concerns About Ectogenesis', *Hypatia* 4, no. 3 (1989): 68.

31 Ibid., 77.

32 Ibid., 75.

33 Claire Horn, 'A History of Gestation Outside the Body', *Wellcome Collection*, 30 November 2021 Accessed 31 January 2025. https://wellcomecollection.org/stories/a-history-of-gestation-outside-the-body

34 Claire Horn, 'Artificial Wombs, Frozen Embryos, and Parenthood: Will Ectogenesis Redistribute Gendered Responsibility for Gestation?' *Feminist Legal Studies* 30 (2022): 51.

35 Gena Corea, *The Mother Machine: Reproductive Technologies from Artificial Insemination to Artificial Wombs* (New York: Harper & Row, 1985).

36 Barbara Katz Rothman, *A Bun in the Oven: How the Food and Birth Movements Resist Industrialization* (New York: NYU Press, 2016), 61.

37 Robyn Rowland, 'Technology and Motherhood: Reproductive Choice Reconsidered.' *Signs* 12, no. 3 (1987): 517.

38 Andrea Dworkin, *Right-Wing Women* (New York: Coward-McCann, 1983), 187–8.

39 Jan Zimmerman, 'Technology and the Future of Women: Haven't We Met Somewhere Before?' *Women's Studies International Forum* 4, no. 3 (1981): 364.

40 Ibid., 365.

41 Farquhar, *The Other Machine*, 22.

42 Mary Anne Case, 'Feminist Fundamentalism as an Individual and Constitutional Commitment', *American University Journal of Gender, Social Policy and the Law* 9, no. 2 (2011): 550.

43 Ibid., 551.

44 Peter Singer and Deane Wells, 'Ectogenesis', in *Ectogenesis: Artificial Womb Technology and the Future of Human Reproduction*, Scott Gelfand and John Shook (eds) (New York: Rodopi, 2006), 9–26.

45 Ibid., 19–20.

46 Anna Smajdor, 'The Moral Imperative for Ectogenesis', *Cambridge Quarterly Healthcare Ethics* 16, no. 3 (2007): 336–45; 'In Defense of Ectogenesis', 90–103.

47 Ibid., 341.

48 Brenda Russell, Debra Oswald and MaryKate Cotter, 'What Makes a Liberal Feminist? Identifying Predictors of Heterosexual Women and Men's Liberal Feminist Ideology', *Analyses of Social Issues and Public Policy* 24, no. 1 (2024): 241.

49 Clare Chambers, 'Introduction: A Feminist Liberalism', in *Freedom and Equality: Essays on Liberalism and Feminism* (Oxford, Oxford University Press, 2024), 1.

50 Amy R. Baehr, 'Liberal Feminism', in *The Stanford Encyclopedia of Philosophy*, Edward N. Zalta (ed.), 2021. Accessed 31 January 2025. https://plato.stanford.edu/archives/spr2021/entries/feminism-liberal

51 Julinna C. Oxley, 'Liberal Feminism', in *Just the Arguments: 100 of the Most Important Arguments in Western Philosophy*, Michael Bruce and Steven Barbone (eds) (Chichester: Blackwell Publishing, 2011), 259.

52 Susan M. Squier, *Babies in Bottles: Twentieth-Century Visions of Reproductive Technology* (New Brunswick: Rutgers University Press, 1994).

53 Sherryl Vint, 'Introduction: Science Fiction and Biopolitics', *Science Fiction Film and Television* 4, no. 2 (2011): 161–72.

54 Lyman Tower Sargent, 'Authority and Utopia: Utopianism in Political Thought', *Polity Journal* 14, no. 4 (1982): 566.

1 Locating ectogenesis

1 Leslie Cannold, 'Women, Ectogenesis and Ethical Theory', *Journal of Applied Philosophy* 12, no. 1 (1995): 55.

2 Jutta Arens, et al., 'NeonatOx: A Pumpless Extracorporeal Lung Support for Premature Neonates', *Artificial Organs* 35, no. 11 (2011): 1000.

3 Emily A. Partridge, et al., 'An Extra-Uterine System to Physiologically Support the Extreme Premature Lamb', *Nature Communications* 8 (2017). DOI: 10.1038/ncomms15112.

4 Ibid.

5 Max Kozlov, 'Human Trials of Artificial Wombs Could Start Soon. Here's What You Need to Know', *Nature*, 14 September 2023. Accessed 22 January 2024. https://www.nature.com/articles/d41586-023-02901-1

6 Aakash M. Shah, 'FDA on the Verge of Approving Human Clinical Trial for Artificial Womb', *Artificial Organs* 47 (2023): 1683–4.
7 Philip Hunter, 'Exogestation for Treating Premature Births and Congenital Diseases: Artificial Womb Technology Edges Toward First Trials in Humans', *EMBO Reports* 25, no. 1 (2024): 17.
8 Haruo Usada, et al., 'Successful Maintenance of Key Physiological Parameters in Preterm Lambs Treated with Ex Vivo Uterine Environment Therapy for a Period of 1 Week', *American Journal of Obstetrics and Gynecology* 217, no. 4 (2017): 457.
9 Elizabeth Chloe Romanis, 'Artificial Womb Technology and Clinical Translation: Innovative Treatment or Medical Research?' *Bioethics* 34, no. 4 (2020): 392.
10 Alan W. Flake, quoted in Rachel Becker, 'An Artificial Womb Successfully Grew Baby Sheep – and Humans Could Be Next', *The Verge*, 25 April 2017. Accessed 22 November 2017. https://www.theverge.com/2017/4/25/15421734/artificial-womb-fetus-biobag-uterus-lamb-sheep-birth-premie-preterm-infant.
11 P. Chavatte-Palmer, R. Lévy and P. Boileau, 'Une Reproduction Sans Utérus? État des Lieux de L'ectogenèse' (Reproduction without a Uterus? State of the Art of Ectogenesis), *Gynécologie Obstétrique and Fertilité* 40, no. 11 (2012): 695.
12 Jessica H. Schultz, 'Development of Ectogenesis: How Will Artificial Wombs Affect the Legal Status of a Fetus or Embryo?' *Chicago-Kent Law Review* 84 (2010): 880.
13 Ibid., 879; Carlo Bulletti, et al., 'The Artificial Womb', *Annals of the New York Academy of Science* 1221 (2011): 125.
14 Schultz, 'Development of Ectogenesis', 880.
15 Braxton Forde, et al., 'Creation of a Novel Synthetic Amniotic Fluid for Use in Fetal Therapy with In-Vitro Testing on Human Amniotic Membranes', *American Journal of Obstetrics and Gynecology MFM* 5, no. 9 (2023): 101055.
16 Nicola Davis, 'Artificial Womb: Dutch Researchers Given €2.9m to Develop Prototype', *The Guardian*, 8 October 2019. Accessed 4 October 2021. https://www.theguardian.com/society/2019/oct/08/artificial-womb-dutch-researchers-given-29m-to-develop-prototype.
17 Anonymous, 'Without Gasping for Air Safely in the Artificial Womb', *TU/e News and Events*, 7 April 2022. Accessed 22 January 2024. https://www.tue.nl/en/storage/biomedische-technologie/de-faculteit/news-and-events/news-overview/07-04-2022-without-gasping-for-air-safely-in-the-artificial-womb.
18 Elselijn Kingma and Suki Finn, 'Neonatal Incubator or Artificial Womb? Distinguishing Ectogestation and Ectogenesis Using the Metaphysics of Pregnancy', *Bioethics* 34, no. 4 (2020): 354–63.
19 Felix De Bie, et al., 'Ethics Considerations Regarding Artificial Womb Technology for the Fetonate', *American Journal of Bioethics* 23, no. 5 (2023): 67–78.

20 M. Verrips, et al., 'Clinical Aspects of Umbilical Cord Cannulation During Transfer from the Uterus to a Liquid-Based Perinatal Life Support System for Extremely Premature Infants: A Qualitative Generic Study', *PLoS One* 18, no. 12 (2023): e0290659.

21 De Bie et al., 'Ethics Considerations Regarding Artificial Womb Technology for the Fetonate', 72–3.

22 Mark R. Mercurio and Kelly M. Werner, 'Thinking Inside the Bag: Patient Selection, Framing the Ethical Discourse, and the Importance of Terminology in Artificial Womb Technology', *American Journal of Bioethics* 23, no. 5 (2023): 79.

23 Nobuya Unno, et al., 'Development of an Artificial Placenta: Survival of Isolated Goat Fetuses for Three Weeks with Umbilical Arteriovenous Extracorporeal Membrane Oxygenation', *Artificial Organs* 17, no. 12 (1993): 1002.

24 Nick Otway and Megan Ellis, 'Construction and Test of an Artificial Uterus for Ex Situ Development of Shark Embryos', *Zoo Biology* 31, no. 2 (2012): 197–205.

25 John Platt, 'Artificial Uterus Could Save Grey Nurse Shark from Extinction', *Scientific American*, 18 February 2009. Accessed 22 January 2024. https://blogs.scientificamerican.com/extinction-countdown/artificial-uterus-could-save-grey-nurse-shark-from-extinction/

26 Corey Binns, 'The Shark Factory: An Artificial Uterus Gives an Endangered Species a Shot at Survival', *Popular Science* 275, no. 1 (2009): 34.

27 Taketeru Tomita, et al., 'Portable-Sized Artificial Uterine System for Viviparous Shark Embryos', *MethodsX* 13 (2024): 103063.

28 J. S. van Haren, et al., 'Simulation-Based Development: Shaping Clinical Procedures for Extra-Uterine Life Support Technology', *Advances in Simulation* 8, no. 29 (2023): DOI: 10.1186/s41077-023-00267-y.

29 Susan Rae Peterson, 'The Politics of Prenatal Diagnosis: A Feminist Ethical Analysis', in *The Custom-Made Child? Women-Centred Perspectives*, Helen B. Holmes, et al. (eds) (New Jersey: Humana Press Inc., 1981), 103.

30 Mary O'Brien, *The Politics of Reproduction* (London: Routledge & Kegan Paul, 1981), 8.

31 Simone de Beauvoir, *The Second Sex*, Constance Borde and Sheila Malovany-Chevallier (trans) (London: Vintage Books, 2010), 567.

32 Janice G. Raymond, 'Maternal Environments and Ejaculatory Fathers: New Definitions of Motherhood and Fatherhood', in *Women as Wombs: Reproductive Technologies and the Battle over Women's Freedom* (Melbourne: Spinifex Press Pty., 1994), 65.

33 Ibid., 68.

34 A number of historical examples can be found here: Jeanne Stellman and Mary Sue Henifin, 'No Fertile Women Need Apply: Employment Discrimination and Reproductive Hazards in the Workplace', in *Biological Woman – The Convenient*

Myth: A Collection of Feminist Essays and a Comprehensive Bibliography, Ruth Hubbard, Mary Sue Henifin and Barbara Fried (eds) (Cambridge: Schenkman Publishing, 1982), 117–20.

35 M. Jean Heriot, 'Fetal Rights versus the Female Body: Contested Domains', *Medical Anthropology Quarterly* 10, no. 2 (1996): 179.

36 Cynthia R. Daniels, 'Fathers, Mothers, and Fetal Harm: Rethinking Gender Difference and Reproductive Responsibility', in *Fetal Subjects, Feminist Positions*, Lynn M. Morgan and Meredith W. Michaels (eds) (Philadelphia: University of Pennsylvania Press, 1999), 83–4. Daniels also notes that environmental exposures such as lead paint and drug use can also be partially attributed to public institutions and social structures and that although responsibility for these are 'deeply shared with men', assumptions about women's role in reproduction has led to an exaggeration of 'maternal mediated risk.'

37 Ronald Dworkin, *Life's Dominion: An Argument about Abortion, Euthanasia and Individual Freedom* (London: Harper Collins, 1993), 160.

38 Jennifer Smookler, 'Feminism, Liberal Democracy and the Politics of Inclusion and Exclusion', *Political Studies Association – UK Annual Conference Proceedings*, University of London (2000): 2.

39 Christine Overall, *Ethics and Human Reproduction: A Feminist Analysis* (London: Routledge, 1987), 167.

40 Danielle Nierenberg, 'The Health Hazards of Being Female', in *Correcting Gender Myopia: Gender Equity, Women's Welfare, and the Environment* (Washington: World Watch Institute, 2002), 37.

41 O'Brien, *The Politics of Reproduction*, 52.

42 This is not to imply they are excluded from family creation via other means.

43 Kendal, *Equal Opportunity and the Case for State Sponsored Ectogenesis*, 27.

44 Jeffery P. Baker, 'The Incubator and the Medical Discovery of the Premature Infant', *Journal of Perinatalogy* 5 (2000): 321–8; Jeffery P. Baker, 'The Incubator Controversy: Pediatricians and the Origins of Premature Infant Technology in the United States, 1890 to 1910', *Pediatrics* 87, no. 5 (1991): 654–62.

45 William A. Silverman, 'Incubator-Baby Side Shows,' *Pediatrics* 64, no. 2 (1979): 128.

46 Anil K. Dubey, *Infertility: Diagnosis, Management, & IVF* (New Delhi: Jaypee Brothers Medical Publishers, 2012), 17.

47 Giuseppe Benagiano, et al., 'Robert G Edwards and the Roman Catholic Church,' *Reproductive Biomedicine Online* 22 (2011): 670.

48 John D. Biggers, 'IVF and Embryo Transfer: Historical Origin and Development', *Reproductive Biomedicine Online* 25, no. 2 (2012): 119.

49 Aldous Huxley, *Brave New World* (London: Chatto and Windus, 1932).

50 Squier, *Babies in Bottles*, 67.

51 Jay Clayton, 'The Ridicule of Time: Science Fiction, Bioethics, and the Posthuman,' *American Literary History* 25, no. 2 (2013): 318.

52 Sarah DiGregorio, 'Artificial Wombs Aren't a Sci-Fi Horror Story', *Slate*, 30 January 2020. Accessed 22 January 2024. https://slate.com/technology/2020/01/artificial-wombs-science-fiction-pregnancy-premature.html

53 De Bie et al., 'Ethics Considerations Regarding Artificial Womb Technology for the Fetonate', 67–78.

54 Ibid., 68.

55 Partridge et al., 'An Extra-Uterine System to Physiologically Support the Extreme Premature Lamb', 15112.

56 De Bie et al., 'Ethics Considerations Regarding Artificial Womb Technology for the Fetonate', 67.

57 Ibid., 74.

58 Seppe Segers and Dorian Accoe, 'The Ethics of Ectogestative Technology – Telling Science from Science Fiction', *JAMA Pediatrics* 177, no. 10 (2023): 1110.

59 Ibid.

60 Tessa Gavina et al., 'Artificial Wombs or Artificial Feminism: What Is Wrong with Being Pregnant?' *American Journal of Bioethics* 23, no. 5 (2023): 104.

61 Singer and Wells, 'Ectogenesis', 22.

62 Schultz, 'Development of Ectogenesis', 894. Amed Alghrani and Margaret Brazier also suggest that benefit to *future* foetuses might be sufficient ethical grounds to enroll some current premature infants in experimentation trials. Amed Alghrani and Margaret Brazier 'What Is It? Whose It? Re-positioning the Fetus in the Context of Research?' *Cambridge Law Journal* 70, no. 1 (2011): 70.

63 Mercurio and Werner, 'Thinking Inside the Bag', 80.

64 Ibid., 79–80.

65 Ibid., 79.

66 E. J. (Joanne) Verweij and Elselijn Kingma, 'Artificial Placenta – Imminent Ethical Considerations for Research Trials and Clinical Translation', *American Journal of Bioethics* 23, no. 5 (2023): 86.

67 Ibid.

68 Ibid.

69 John D. Lantos and Annie Janvier, 'The Dilemmas of Artificial Wombs: Conventional Ethics and Science Fiction', *American Journal of Bioethics* 23, no. 5 (2023): 82.

70 Montserrat Esquerda, et al., 'Beyond the Domains: What Would be the Fundamental Ethical Questions in the Development of the Artificial Womb', *American Journal of Bioethics* 23, no. 5 (2023): 126.

71 Stephanie K. Kukora, George B. Mychaliska and Elliott Mark Weiss, 'Ethical Challenges for First-in-Human Trials of the Artificial Placenta and Artificial

Womb: Not All Technologies are Created Equally, Ethically', *Journal of Perinatology* 43 (2023): 1337–42.

72 Mercurio and Werner, 'Thinking Inside the Bag', 80.

73 Ibid.

74 Ibid.

75 Esquerda, et al., 'Beyond the Domains', 125.

76 James J. Cordeiro, 'On the Permissibility of Elective Ectogestation', *American Journal of Bioethics* 23, no. 5 (2023): 116.

77 John Holmes and Laura Hosford, 'Artificial Womb Technology, Catholic Health Care, and Social Justice', *American Journal of Bioethics* 23, no. 5 (2023): 123–5.

78 Christopher Kaczor, 'Artificial Wombs and Embryo Adoption', in *The Ethics of Embryo Adoption and the Catholic Tradition: Moral Arguments, Economic Reality and Social Analysis*, Sarah-Vaughan Brakman and Darlene Fozard Weaver (eds) (Dordrecht: Springer, 2007), 307–22.

79 Holmes and Hosford, 'Artificial Womb Technology, Catholic Health Care, and Social Justice',123–4.

80 Muhammad Ahmad Ibrahim AlJahsh, 'Science and Islamic Ethics: Navigating Artificial Womb Technology Through Quranic Principles', *Heliyon* 10 (2024): e36793.

81 Marcia C. Inhorn, *Local Babies, Global Science: Gender, Religion and In Vitro Fertilization in Egypt* (New York: Routledge, 2003).

82 De Bie, et al., 'Ethics Considerations Regarding Artificial Womb Technology for the Fetonate', 73.

83 Ibid.

84 Tamara Kayali Browne, Evie Kendal and Tiia Sudenkaarne, 'Feminist Concerns About Artificial Womb Technology', *American Journal of Bioethics* 23, no. 5 (2023): 98.

85 Seppe Segers, Guido Pennings and Heidi Mertens, 'The Ethics of Ectogenesis-aided Foetal Treatment', *Bioethics* 34 (2020): 367.

86 Browne et al. 'Feminist Concerns About Artificial Womb Technology', 98.

87 Ibid.

88 Seppe Segers and Elizabeth Chloe Romanis, 'Ethical, Translational, and Legal Issues Surrounding the Novel Adoption of Ectogestative Technologies', *Risk Management and Healthcare Policy* 15 (2022): 2207.

89 Verweij and Kingma, 'Artificial Placenta', 85.

90 Ibid.

91 Susan Kennedy and Lawrence Nelson, 'A Different Take on the Law and Ethics of AWT', *American Journal of Bioethics* 23, no. 5 (2023): 93.

92 Ibid.

93 United States Supreme Court, *Roe v. Wade,* 410 U.S. 113 (1973) enshrined federal abortion rights in the United States of America for almost 50 years based on a Constitutional right to privacy. Protections were dependent on the gestational age of the foetus, with increasing State interest in foetal life recognized the further the pregnancy progressed. When this ruling was overturned, it allowed individual States to regulate abortion, with some severely restricting access. All States are still bound by the federal Emergency Medical Treatment and Active Labor Act (1986) (EMTALA) to provide abortions if the pregnant person's life is in danger and terminating the pregnancy would help stabilize the patient (United States Department of Health and Human Services Office of the Inspector General. 'The Emergency Medical Treatment and Labor Act (EMTALA).' November 2024. Accessed 30 January 2025. https://oig.hhs.gov/reports-and-publications/featured-topics/emtala/).

94 Monika Jordan, 'The Post-Dobbs World: How the Implementation of Fetal Personhood Laws Will Affect In Vitro Fertilization', *UIC Law Review* 57, no. 2 (2024): 257.

95 Kennedy and Nelson, 'A Different Take on the Law and Ethics of AWT', 94.

96 In February 2024, the US State of Alabama in *LePage v Center for Reproductive Medicine* declared frozen embryos as 'children' for whom wrongful death claims could be made, effectively halting IVF procedures in the State, *see* Lauren Mascarenhas and Melissa Alonso, 'Alabama State Senator Proposes Bill to Protect IVF Medical Providers', *CNN*, 27 February 2024. Accessed 28 February 2024. https://edition.cnn.com/2024/02/27/us/ivf-ruling-impact-other-states/index.html; Edward R. Grant, 'The Short-Lived Verdict in *Le Page v Center for Reproductive Medicine*: Why "Personhood" Matters in the Regulation of Assisted Reproductive Technologies', *Medical Law Review* 32 (2024): 399–409. If such rulings persist, failure to use ectogenesis if available may one day also carry penalties.

97 Elizabeth Chloe Romanis, 'The Ethical and Legal Status of "Fetonates" or "Gestatelings"', *American Journal of Bioethics* 23, no. 5 (2023): 90–92; Elizabeth Chloe Romanis, 'Artificial Womb Technology and the Significance of Birth: Why Gestatelings Are Not Newborns (or Fetuses)', *Journal of Medical Ethics* 45, no. 11 (2019): 728–31.

98 Lien De Proost and Geertjan Zuijdwegt, 'Lost in Gestation: On Fetonates, Perinates, and Gestatelings', *American Journal of Bioethics* 23, no. 5 (2023): 108.

99 Ibid., 109.

100 Ibid., 110.

101 Ibid.

102 Verweij and Kingma, 'Artificial Placenta', 85.

103 De Bie, et al., 'Ethics Considerations Regarding Artificial Womb Technology for the Fetonate', 74.

104 Kingma and Finn, 'Neonatal Incubator or Artificial Womb?' 354–63.
105 Romanis, 'The Ethical and Legal Status of "Fetonates" or "Gestatelings"', 90.
106 Ibid.
107 Elizabeth Chloe Romanis, 'Challenging the "Born Alive" Threshold: Fetal Surgery, Artificial Wombs, and the English Approach to Legal Personhood', *Medical Law Review* 28, no. 1 (2020): 93–123.
108 Esquerda, et al., 'Beyond the Domains', 125–6.
109 Ibid., 126.
110 It should be noted here that concerns about the moral significance of birth for attaining legal rights are not new, with Mary Anne Warren's 1989 article on abortion considering similar issues to those seen here regarding ectogenesis; *see* Mary Anne Warren, 'The Moral Significance of Birth', *Hypatia* 4, no. 3 (1989): 46–65.
111 Leonard Michael Fleck, 'Abortion, Artificial Wombs, and the "No Difference" Argument', *American Journal of Bioethics* 23, no. 5 (2023): 95.
112 Romanis, 'The Ethical and Legal Status of "Fetonates" Or "Gestatelings"', 91.
113 De Proost and Zuijdwegt, 'Lost in Gestation', 109–10.
114 Kennedy and Nelson, 'A Different Take on the Law and Ethics of AWT', 93.
115 Mercurio and Werner, 'Thinking Inside the Bag', 81.
116 De Proost and Zuijdwegt, 'Lost in Gestation', 109.
117 Judith Jarvis Thomson, 'A Defense of Abortion', *Philosophy and Public Affairs* 1, no. 1 (1971): 47–66. Here, as an analogy for pregnancy, Thomson imagines an unsuspecting individual has been kidnapped and wakes up to find they have been hooked up to a famous violinist who suffers a kidney condition and temporarily requires the victim's kidneys to filter toxins from their bloodstream. She argues that the individual retains the right to disconnect themselves even though this will lead to the death of the violinist and regardless of the fact the violinist only needs this life support system for a fixed period of time.
118 Eric Steiger, 'Not of Woman Born: How Ectogenesis Will Change the Way We View Viability, Birth, and the Status of the Unborn', *Journal of Law and Health* 23 (2010): 146.
119 De Proost and Zuijdwegt, 'Lost in Gestation', 109.
120 This argument is sometimes referred to as 'severance theory' and commits its adherents to support methods of termination of pregnancy that would not necessarily bring about the death of the foetus, potentially including foetal extraction and subsequent artificial gestation.
121 Steiger, 'Not of Woman Born', 14.
122 Joan C. Callahan and James W. Knight, 'Women, Fetuses, Medicine, and the Law', in *Feminist Perspectives in Medical Ethics*, Helen Bequaert Holmes and Laura M. Purdy (eds.) (USA: Indiana University Press, 1992), 231.

123 Claire Horn, 'Ectogenesis Is for Feminists: Reclaiming Artificial Wombs from Anti-abortion Discourse', *Catalyst: Feminism, Theory, Technoscience* 6, no. 1 (2020): 5.
124 Browne et al., 'Feminist Concerns About Artificial Womb Technology', 98.
125 Nina Roesner, 'Beyond a Medicalized View of Reproduction: Recentering Pregnant People in the Ethics of Ectogenesis', *American Journal of Bioethics* 23, no. 5 (2023): 103.
126 Joona Räsänen, 'Ectogenesis, Abortion and a Right to the Death of the Fetus', *Bioethics* 31, no. 9 (2017): 697.
127 Cannold, 'Women, Ectogenesis and Ethical Theory', 61.
128 Seppe Segers, 'The Path Toward Ectogenesis: Looking Beyond the Technical Challenges', *BMC Medical Ethics* 22 (2021): 59.
129 Benjamin Patterson Brown and Katie Watson, 'No Substitute: The False Promise of Artificial Womb Technology as an Alternative to Abortion', *American Journal of Bioethics* 23, no. 5 (2023): 88.
130 Ibid., 88–9.
131 Ibid., 88.
132 Fleck, 'Abortion, Artificial Wombs, and the "No Difference" Argument', 96.
133 Ibid.
134 Ibid., 95.
135 Ibid.
136 De Bie, et al., 'Ethics Considerations Regarding Artificial Womb Technology for the Fetonate', 73.
137 Matteo Gulino, et al., 'Artificial Womb on Maternal Request and without the Father's Consent: Ethical Perspectives Through a Principlist Approach', *American Journal of Bioethics* 23, no. 5 (2023): 121.
138 Ibid., 121–2.
139 Ibid., 122.
140 Kyoko Takashima, et al., 'Is the Mother's Decision to Opt for Artificial Womb Technology Always "Supererogatory"?' *American Journal of Bioethics* 23, no. 5 (2023): 119–20.
141 Ibid., 120.
142 Steiger, 'Not of Woman Born', 159–60.
143 Fleck, 'Abortion, Artificial Wombs, and the "No Difference" Argument', 95.
144 Gulino, et al., 'Artificial Womb on Maternal Request and without the Father's Consent', 122.
145 Ibid.
146 Tim Bayne and Avery Kolers, 'Towards a Pluralist Account of Parenthood', *Bioethics* 17, no. 3 (2003): 238.
147 Browne et al., 'Feminist Concerns About Artificial Womb Technology', 97.

148 Ibid.

149 Ibid.

150 Roesner, 'Beyond a Medicalized View of Reproduction', 102; Leah Lomotey-Nakon and Elizabeth Lanphier, 'Expanding the Frame: An Afrofuturist Response to Artificial Womb Technology', *American Journal of Bioethics* 23, no. 5 (2023): 100; Laura L. Kimberly and Gwendolyn P. Quinn, 'Toward a Broader Conception of Equity in Artificial Womb Technology', *American Journal of Bioethics* 23, no. 5 (2023): 114.

151 Gavina et al., 'Artificial Wombs or Artificial Feminism', 105.

152 Ibid.

153 Roesner, 'Beyond a Medicalized View of Reproduction', 103.

154 Ibid.

155 Kimberly and Quinn, 'Toward a Broader Conception of Equity in Artificial Womb Technology', 115.

156 Ibid.

157 Ibid.

158 Ibid.

159 Gavina et al., 'Artificial Wombs or Artificial Feminism', 105; Kimberly and Quinn, 'Toward a Broader Conception of Equity in Artificial Womb Technology', 114.

160 Lomotey-Nakon and Lanphier, 'Expanding the Frame', 101; Lantos and Janvier, 'The Dilemmas of Artificial Wombs', 84.

161 Mercurio and Werner, 'Thinking Inside the Bag', 80.

162 Ibid.; Esquerda, et al., 'Beyond the Domains', 126.

163 Anonymous, 'In Vitro', *Space' Above and Beyond* wiki, 11 July 2017. Accessed 5 February 2024. https://spaceaboveandbeyond.fandom.com/wiki/In_Vitro

164 Roesner, 'Beyond a Medicalized View of Reproduction', 102.

165 Ibid.

166 David Weber, *At All Costs* (Riverdale, NY: Baen Books, 2005), 105.

167 Lois McMaster Bujold. *Shards of Honor* (New York: Baen Books, 1986).

168 Fekade Getachew Hailu, et al., 'Advanced Abdominal Pregnancy, with Live Fetus and Severe Preeclampsia, Case Report', *BMC Pregnancy and Childbirth* 17 (2017): 243. It should be noted these authors suggest claims of viable abdominal pregnancies should be considered with a 'high index of suspicion' due to the extreme rarity of such events.

169 This would also require revisions to various laws restricting embryo experimentation beyond 14 days' development; *see* ACOG, 'Preembryo Research History, Scientific Background, and Ethical Considerations', *International Journal of Gynaecology and Obstetrics* 45 (1994): 291–301.

170 Bayne and Kolers, 'Towards a Pluralist Account of Parenthood', 238.

171 Lomotey-Nakon and Lanphier, 'Expanding the Frame', 100.

172 Ibid., 100–101.

173 Lantos and Janvier, 'The Dilemmas of Artificial Wombs', 84.
174 Ibid.

2 The role of imagination in bioethics

1 Alan R. White, *The Language of Imagination* (Oxford: Basil Blackwell, 1990), 5.
2 Ibid.
3 René Descartes, *The Philosophical Writings of Descartes, Volume III: The Correspondence*, John Cottingham et al. (trans) (Cambridge: Cambridge University Press, 1991), 186.
4 George Berkeley, *The Works of George Berkeley, Bishop of Cloyne*, Volume 2, A. A. Luce and T. E. Jessop (eds) (London: Nelson, 1948), 8–9 [editorial comment].
5 Martin Jay, 'In the Realm of the Senses: An Introduction', *American Historical Review* 116, no. 2 (2011): 310.
6 Paul Lauritzen, 'Visual Bioethics', *American Journal of Bioethics* 8, no. 12 (2008): 50.
7 Ibid.
8 White, *The Language of Imagination*, 44.
9 Fiona Hughes, *Kant's Critique of Aesthetic Judgement* (London: Continuum, 2010), 21.
10 'Imagination', in *A Wittgenstein Dictionary*, Hans-Johann Glock (ed.), *Blackwell Reference Online*, 1996, DOI: 10.1111/b.9780631185376.1996.x.
11 Alfred Nordmann, *Wittgenstein's Tractatus: An Introduction* (Cambridge: Cambridge University Press, 2005), 170.
12 White, *The Language of Imagination*, 184.
13 Istvan Csicsery-Ronay, Jr., *The Seven Beauties of Science Fiction* (Connecticut: Wesleyan University Press, 2008), 2–3.
14 Sheryl N. Hamilton, 'Traces of the Future: Biotechnology, Science Fiction, and the Media', *Science Fiction Studies* 30, no. 2 (2003): 269.
15 Ibid.
16 Lauritzen, 'Visual Bioethics', 50.
17 Ibid.
18 Ibid., 51, 54.
19 Catherine Mills, 'Images and Emotion in Abortion Debates', *American Journal of Bioethics* 8, no. 12 (2008): 61.
20 Kathryn Woodward, 'Introduction to Part Three', in *The Gendered Cyborg: A Reader*, Gill Kirkup, Kathryn Woodward and Fiona Hovenden (eds) (London: Routledge, 2000), 164.
21 Rosalind Pollack Petchesky, 'Fetal Images: The Power of Visual Culture in the Politics of Reproduction', *Feminist Studies* 13, no. 2 (1987): 263–4.

22 Ibid.
23 Ibid., 268.
24 Suzanne Anker and Sarah Franklin, 'Specimens as Spectacles: Reframing Fetal Remains', *Social Texts* 29, no. 1 (2011): 116.
25 Woodward, 'Introduction to Part Three', 164–5.
26 Barbara Duden, *The Woman Beneath the Skin: A Doctor's Patients in Eighteenth-Century Germany*, Thomas Dunlap (trans) (Cambridge: Harvard University Press, 1991), 170.
27 Susan Squier, 'Negotiating Boundaries: From Assisted Reproduction to Assisted Replication', in *Playing Dolly: Technocultural Formations, Fantasies, & Fictions of Assisted Reproduction*, E. Ann Kaplan and Susan Squier (eds) (New Brunswick: Rutgers University Press, 1999), 104.
28 Heather Latimer, 'Reproductive Technologies, Fetal Icons, and Genetic Freaks: Shelley Jackson's *Patchwork Girl* and the Limits and Possibilities of Donna Haraway's Cyborg', *Modern Fiction Studies* 57, no. 2 (2011): 319.
29 Lynn M. Morgan and Meredith W. Michaels, 'Part II: Manipulating the Fetal Image', in *Fetal Subjects, Feminist Positions*, Lynn M. Morgan and Meredith W. Michaels (eds) (Philadelphia: University of Pennsylvania Press, 1999), 99.
30 Farquhar, *The Other Machine*, 163.
31 Niamh Stephenson, Catherine Mills and Kim McLeod, '"Simply Providing Information": Negotiating the Ethical Dilemmas of Obstetric Ultrasound, Prenatal Testing and Selective Termination of Pregnancy', *Feminism and Psychology* 27, no. 1 (2016): 73.
32 *The Island*, [Film] directed by Michael Bay (California: DreamWorks Pictures, 2005).
33 J.B.S. Haldane, *Daedalus: or, Science and the Future: A Paper Read to the Heretics, Cambridge, on February 4th, 1923* (London: Kegan Paul, Trench, Trubner, 1924), 44.
34 Nick Bostrom, 'A History of Transhumanist Thought', *Journal of Evolution & Technology* 14, no. 1 (2005): 4.
35 Sara Ahmed, 'The Performativity of Disgust', in *The Cultural Politics of Emotion* (New York and London: Routledge, 2004), 85.
36 *The Matrix*, [Film] directed by Lana and Lilly Wachowski (Burbank, California: Warner Bros., 1999).
37 Leon R. Kass, 'The Wisdom of Repugnance', *New Republic* 216, no. 22 (1997): 20.
38 Ibid.
39 Lauritzen, 'Visual Bioethics', 51.
40 Julia Kristeva, *Powers of Horror: An Essay on Abjection*, Leon S. Roudiez (trans) (New York: Columbia University Press, 1982), 4.
41 Ibid., 70.

42 Philip Ball, *Unnatural: The Heretical Idea of Making People* (London: The Bodley Head, 2011), 189.
43 Northrop Frye, *On Education* (Ontario: Fitzhenry & Whiteside, 1988), 54
44 Lisa Cartwright, *Moral Spectatorship: Technologies of Voice and Affect in Postwar Representations of the Child* (Durham: Duke University Press, 2008), 56.
45 Evelyn Tsitas, 'The Role of the Creative Arts in Bioethical Debates', *Law and Justice Journal* 6, no. 2 (2006): 260.
46 Sheila Jasanoff, 'Future Imperfect: Science, Technology, and the Imaginations of Modernity', in *Dreamscapes of Modernity: Sociotechnical Imaginaries and the Fabrication of Power*, Sheila Jasanoff and Kim Sang-Hyun (eds) (Chicago: University of Chicago Press, 2015), 3.
47 Ibid., 1.
48 Colin Radford and Michael Weston, 'How Can We Be Moved by the Fate of Anna Karenina?' *Proceedings of the Aristotelian Society, Supplementary Volumes* 49 (1975): 70.
49 Ibid., 71.
50 Daniel Jacobson, 'Sir Philip Sydney's Dilemma: On the Ethical Treatment of Narrative Art', *Journal of Aesthetics and Art Criticism* 54, no. 4 (1996): 327.
51 Ibid., 333.
52 Ibid., 334.
53 Noël Carroll, 'The Wheel of Virtue: Art, Literature, and Moral Knowledge', *Journal of Aesthetics and Art Criticism* 60, no. 1 (2002): 9.
54 Ibid.
55 Kincaid, 'On the Origins of Genre', 409.
56 Andrew Milner, *Literature, Culture and Society*, 2nd edition (London: Routledge, 2004), 137; Mary Shelley, *Frankenstein: Or, the Modern Prometheus* (London: Lackington, Hughes, Harding, Mavor & Jones, 1818).
57 Kincaid, 'On the Origins of Genre', 409.
58 Matthew Cheney, 'Science Fiction and Difference: An Introduction to Starboard Wine', in Samuel R. Delany *Starboard Wine: More Notes on the Language of Science Fiction* (Middleton, Connecticut: Wesleyan University Press, 2012), xxiv.
59 Thomas R. Lindloff, Kelly Coyle and Debra Grodin, 'Is There a Text in This Audience? Science Fiction and Interpretive Schism', in *Theorizing Fandom: Fans, Subculture and Identity*, Cheryl Harris and Alison Alexander (eds) (New Jersey: Hampton Press, 1998), 224.
60 Samuel R. Delany, *Starboard Wine: More Notes on the Language of Science Fiction* (Middleton, Connecticut: Wesleyan University Press, 2012), 153.
61 Ibid.
62 John Rieder, 'On Defining SF, or Not: Genre Theory, SF, and History', *Science Fiction Studies* 37, no. 2 (2010): 197.

63 Paul Kincaid, 'On the Origins of Genre', *Extrapolation* 44, no. 4 (2003): 417.
64 Rieder, 'On Defining SF, or Not', 194.
65 Kincaid, 'On the Origins of Genre', 416–17.
66 Rieder, 'On Defining SF, or Not', 194.
67 Andrew Milner, 'Colonialism and the Emergence of Science Fiction by John Rieder (review)', *Science Fiction Film and Television* 6, no. 1 (2013): 141.
68 Rhys Williams goes so far as to label this 'the Suvin event' (Rhys Williams, 'Recognizing Cognition: On Suvin, Miéville, and the Utopian Impulse in the Contemporary Fantastic', *Science Fiction Studies* 41, no. 3 [2014]: 617).
69 Darko Suvin, 'On What Is and Is Not an SF Narration: With a List of 101 Victorian Books That Should Be Excluded from SF Bibliographies', *Science Fiction Studies* 5, no. 1 (1978): 45.
70 Peter Lowentrout, 'The "Metamorphoses" of Darko Suvin: Final Synthesis or Dogged Antithesis?' *Foundation*, no. 42 (1988): 38.
71 Darko Suvin, 'The State of the Art in Science Fiction Theory: Determining and Delimiting the Genre (Etat présent de la théorie de science-fiction: détermination et délimitation du genre)', *Science Fiction Studies* 6, no. 1 (1979): 37.
72 Ibid.; Darko Suvin, 'Centennial Politics: On Jameson on Brecht on Method', *New Left Review*, no. 234 (1999): 127–40.
73 Fredric Jameson, *Brecht and Method* (London: Verso, 1998), 40.
74 Lowentrout, 'The "Metamorphoses" of Darko Suvin', 43.
75 Gregory Renault, 'Science Fiction as Cognitive Estrangement: Darko Suvin and the Marxist Critique of Mass Culture', *Discourse* 2 (1980): 115, 121.
76 Carl Freedman, *Critical Theory and Science Fiction* (Middletown: Wesleyan University Press, 2013), 13, 17.
77 Ibid., 18.
78 Ibid.
79 China Miéville, 'Cognition as Ideology: A Dialectic of SF Theory', in *Red Planets: Marxism and Science Fiction*, Mark Bould and China Miéville (eds) (London: Pluto, 2009), 238.
80 Ibid.
81 Mark Bould, '*Critical Theory and Science Fiction*, Carl Freedman. Hanover: Wesleyan University Press/University Press of New England, 2000 [review]', *Historical Materialism* 10, no. 4 (2002): 300.
82 Benjamin J. Robertson, '*Freedman, Carl. Art and Idea in the Novels of China Miéville*. Canterbury, UK: Gylphi, 2015. 183 pp. Paperback. ISBN 978-1-78024-030-5. $29.99; Edwards, Caroline and Tony Venezia, eds. *China Miéville: Critical Essays*. Canterbury, UK: Gylphi, 2015. 296 pp. Paperback. ISBN 978-1-78024-027-5. $29.99 [review]', *Journal of the Fantastic in the Arts* 27, no. 2 (2016): 365.
83 Williams, 'Recognizing Cognition', 620.

84 Ibid., 621.
85 Freedman, *Critical Theory and Science Fiction*, 19.
86 Suvin, 'On What Is and Is Not an SF Narration', 48 [emphasis mine].
87 Freedman, *Critical Theory and Science Fiction*, 19.
88 Kathleen L. Spencer, '"The Red Sun Is High, the Blue Low": Towards a Stylistic Description of Science Fiction ("Le soleil rouge est au zénith, le soleil bleu se couche": vers une description stylistique de la SF)', *Science Fiction Studies* 10, no. 1 (1983): 36.
89 Ibid., 37.
90 Suvin, 'The State of the Art in Science Fiction Theory', 36; Darko Suvin, 'Narrative Logic, Ideological Domination, and the Range of Science Fiction: A Hypothesis with a Historical Test (Logique narrative, dominate idéologique et l'éventail de la S-F: hypothèse et épreuve historique)', *Science Fiction Studies* 9, no. 1 (1982): 4–5.
91 The Doctor's time machine. TARDIS stands for Time and Relative Dimension in Space.
92 Darko Suvin, 'Defining the Literary Genre of Utopia: Some Historical Semantics, Some Genology, a Proposal and a Plea', *Studies in the Literary Imagination* 6, no. 2 (1973): 144.
93 Peter Fitting, 'Utopia, Dystopia and Science Fiction', in *Cambridge Companion to Utopian Literature*, Gregory Claeys (ed.) (Cambridge: Cambridge University Press, 2010), 147.
94 Alessa Johns, 'Feminism and Utopia', in *The Cambridge Companion to Utopian Literature*, Gregory Claeys (ed.) (Cambridge: Cambridge University Press, 2010), 175.
95 Fátima Vieira, 'The Concept of Utopia', in *The Cambridge Companion to Utopian Literature*, Gregory Claeys (ed.) (Cambridge: Cambridge University Press, 2010), 8.
96 Johns, 'Feminism and Utopia', 174.
97 Ibid., 193.
98 John Rieder, 'Review: Utopia, SF, and the Ideology of Form', *Science Fiction Studies* 42, no. 3 (2015): 566.
99 Sümeyra Buran, 'Being an Artificial Womb Machine-Human', in Sherryl Vint and Sümeyra Buran (eds), *Technologies of Feminist Speculative Fiction: Gender, Artificial Life, and the Politics of Reproduction* (Cham: Palgrave, 2022), 47.
100 Tom Moylan, *Demand the Impossible: Science Fiction and the Utopian Imagination* (London: Methuen, 1986), 2.
101 Brian Garvey, 'Review: The Utopian Imagination', *Science Fiction Studies* 15, no. 2 (1988): 244.
102 Moylan, *Demand the Impossible*, 2.
103 Tom Moylan, *Scraps of the Untainted Sky: Science Fiction, Utopia, Dystopia* (Boulder, Colorado: Westview Press, 2000), 191

104 Greg Claeys, 'The Origins of Dystopia: Wells, Huxley and Orwell', in *The Cambridge Companion to Utopian Literature*, Gregory Claeys (ed.) (Cambridge: Cambridge University Press, 2010), 109.

105 Andrew Milner, 'Resources for a Journey of Hope: Raymond Williams on Utopia and Science Fiction', *Cultural Sociology* 10, no. 4 (2016): 415.

106 The need to return to more liberal and socialist conceptions of science fiction is also evident in light of the current wave of anti-liberal sentiment epitomized by the so-called 'sad puppy' and 'rabid puppy' movements, which under the guise of a return to more conservative science fiction have led to significant personal and professional harassment for those writing feminist science fiction, disproportionately targeting women, and especially women of colour. As such a development can hardly be expected to promote feminist engagement in the genre, a firmly pro-liberal stance is adopted here.

107 Hilde Lindemann Nelson, 'Introduction: How to Do Things with Stories', in *Stories and Their Limits: Narrative Approaches to Bioethics*, Hilde L. Nelson (ed.) (London: Routledge, 1997), x.

108 Ibid.

109 Ibid.

110 Martha C. Nussbaum, '"Finely Aware and Richly Responsible": Literature and the Moral Imagination', in *Love's Knowledge: Essays on Philosophy and Literature* (New York: Oxford University Press, 1990), 148.

111 Nelson, 'Introduction', 153.

112 It should be noted that Nelson also states: 'maybe advanced training in literary theory can, as Nussbaum asserts, make us finely aware and richly responsible. I doubt it, though. I've met literary scholars – and moral philosophers, for that matter – who were complete and utter jerks.' Hilde Lindemann, 'In the Matter of Stories', *Perspectives in Biology and Medicine* 60, no. 1 (2017): 102.

113 Ibid.

114 Ibid., xi.

115 Ibid., xii.

116 Tod Chambers, *The Fiction of Bioethics: Cases as Literary Texts* (New York: Routledge, 1999), 2.

117 Ibid.

118 Ibid., 4.

119 Of interest here is Gérard Genette's theory on paratexts, which states that the addressee of all prefaces is easy to identify as the intended reader of the text (Gérard Genette, 'The Prefactorial Situation of Communication', in *Paratexts: Thresholds of Interpretation* (Cambridge: Cambridge University Press, 2009), 194).

120 K. Danner Clouser, 'Philosophy, Literature, and Ethics: Let the Engagement Begin', *Journal of Medicine and Philosophy* 21 (1996): 335
121 Chambers, *The Fiction of Bioethics*, 176.
122 James F. Childress, 'Case Narratives and Moral Perspectives: An Appreciative Response to Chambers', *American Journal of Bioethics* 1, no. 1 (2001): 58.
123 Ibid.
124 James S. Terry and Peter C. Williams, 'Literature and Bioethics: The Tension in Goals and Styles', *Literature and Medicine* 7 (1988): 5.
125 Valentina Adami, *Bioethics Through Literature: Margaret Atwood's Cautionary Tales* (Trier: Wissenschaftlicher Verlag Trier, 2011), 39.
126 Valentina Adami, 'Between Bioethics and Literature: Representations of (Post) human Identities in Margaret Atwood's Oryx and Crake and The Year of the Flood', *Polemos: Journal of Law, Literature and Culture* 6, no. 2 (2012): 250–1.

3 Science fiction engaging with bioethics

1 Robert Edwards, *Life Before Birth: Reflections on the Embryo Debate* (London: Hutchinson, 1989), 86.
2 Ibid, 92.
3 Ibid.
4 Milner, *Literature, Culture and Society*, 137.
5 Patrick Steptoe interview in *Times*, April 4, 1988, cited in Elizabeth Webber and Mike Feinsilber, *Merriam-Webster's Dictionary of Allusions* (Massachussetts: Merriam-Webster, 1999), 210. Gregory Pence also relates that the scientists involved in the first artificial insemination trials were labelled 'perverts': Gregory Pence, 'What's So Good about Natural Motherhood? (In Praise of Unnatural Gestation)', in *Ectogenesis: Artificial Womb Technology and the Future of Human Reproduction*, Scott Gelfand and John Shook (eds) (New York: Rodopi, 2006), 80.
6 *The Island* (2005).
7 Ibid.
8 *The 6th Day*, [Film] directed by Roger Spottiswoode (California: Sony Pictures, 2000).
9 *The Island* (2005).
10 Arguing for the inevitability of technological development is central to Intel CEO Andy Grove, *Only the Paranoid Survive: How to Exploit the Crisis Points that Challenge Every Company* (New York: Doubleday, 1996) , in which he states: 'In technology, whatever *can* be done *will* be done. We can't stop these changes. We can't hide from them. Instead we must focus on getting ready for them'

(p. 5). Similarly, Daniel Chandler's so-called 'inevitability thesis' also suggests technological development is an irresistible force in 'Technological or Media Determinism' (1995). Available online: http://www.aber.ac.uk/media/Documents/tecdet/tdet01.html

11 Kieran Tranter, 'The Speculative Jurisdiction: The Science Fictionality of Law and Technology', *Griffith Law Review* 20, no. 4 (2011): 826.

12 John Mendeloff, 'Politics and Bioethical Commissions: "Muddling Through" and the "Slippery Slope"', *Journal of Health Politics, Policy and Law* 10, no. 1 (1985): 88.

13 Ibid., 83.

14 Leon Kass, 'Forbidding Science: Some Beginning Reflections', *Science and Engineering Ethics* 15 (2009): 275.

15 Lewis Wolpert, 'The Medawar Lecture 1998: Is Science Dangerous?' *Philosophical Transactions: Biological Sciences* 360, no. 1458 (2005): 1253.

16 Roslynn Haynes, 'From Alchemy to Artificial Intelligence: Stereotypes of the Scientist in Western Literature', *Public Understanding of Science* 12, no. 3 (2003): 243.

17 Ibid.

18 *Splice*, [Film] directed by Vincenzo Natali (Neuilly-sur-Seine, France: Gaumont, 2009).

19 Ibid.

20 Philip J. Nickel, 'Horror and the Idea of Everyday Life: On Skeptical Threats in *Psycho* and *The Birds*', in *The Philosophy of Horror*, Thomas Fahey (ed.) (Kentucky: The University Press of Kentucky, 2010), 18–19.

21 Noël Carroll, *The Philosophy of Horror: Or, Paradoxes of the Heart* (New York: Routledge, 1990), 14.

22 Ibid., 210.

23 National Health and Medical Research Council, 'NHMRC Opens Public Consultation on Draft Ethical Guidelines for Xenotransplantation Research', NHMRC website. Accessed 9 July 2016. https://www.nhmrc.gov.au/media/releases/2016/nhmrc-opens-public-consultation-draft-ethical-guidelines-xenotransplantation.

24 *The X-Files*, 'Emily', [Film] directed by Kim Manners, written by Vince Gilligan, John Shiban and Frank Spotniz (California: Ten Thirteen Productions, 14 December 1997); *The X-files*, 'Essence', [Film] directed by Kim Manners, written by Chris Carter (California: Ten Thirteen Productions, 13 May 2001). *The X-Files* had an initial television run from 1993 to 2002, including nine seasons and a movie in 1998. A second movie was released in 2008, and finally a ten-episode revival (season ten) was released in 2016.

25 Steiger, 'Not of Woman Born', 156.

26 Bayne and Kolers, 'Towards a Pluralist Account of Parenthood', 223.

27 Darko Suvin, *Metamorphoses of Science Fiction: On the Poetics and History of a Literary Genre* (New Haven: Yale University Press, 1979), 81.
28 *Kyle XY*, created by Eric Bress and J. Mackye Gruber (Burbank, California: ABC Studios: 2006–2009).
29 Joseph Millum, 'The Foundation of the Child's Right to an Open Future', *Journal of Social Philosophy* 45, no. 4 (2014): 522–38.
30 Julian Savulescu, 'Procreative Beneficence: Why We Should Select the Best Children', *Bioethics* 15, no. 5–6 (2001): 413–26.
31 William A. W. Walters, 'Cloning, Ectogenesis, and Hybrids: Things to Come?', in *Test-Tube Babies: A Guide to Moral Questions, Present Techniques and Future Possibilities*, William A. W. Walters and Peter Singer (eds) (Melbourne: Oxford University Press, 1982), 116–17.
32 Gina Maranto, *Quest for Perfection: The Drive to Breed Better Human Beings* (New York: Lisa Drew, 1996), 199.
33 Yevgeny Zamyatin, *We* (New York: Modern Library, 2006).
34 Karin Lesnik-Oberstein, *Children's Literature: Criticism and the Fictional Child* (Oxford: Clarendon Press, 1994).
35 Lissa Paul, 'Sex and the Children's Book', *The Lion and the Unicorn* 29, no. 2 (2005): 222.
36 *Fringe*, 'The Same Old Story', [Film] directed by Paul Edwards, written by Jeff Pinkner, J. J. Abrams, Alex Kurtzman and Roberto Orci (Santa Monica: Bad Robot, 16 September 2008).
37 *The Matrix*, [Film] directed by Lana and Lilly Wachowski (Burbank, California: Warner Bros., 1999).
38 Immanuel Kant, 'Groundwork of the Metaphysics of Morals', in *Practical Philosophy*, Mary Gregor (trans) (Cambridge: Cambridge University Press, 1996), 79.
39 Iina Hellsten, 'Popular Metaphors of Biosciences: Bridges Over Time?' *Configurations*, 16, no. 1 (2008): 16.
40 UNESCO, 'Human Dignity and the Human Genome, Article 11', in *Universal Declaration on the Human Genome and Human Rights* (Paris: UNESCO, 1998), 44.
41 Ibid., 42.
42 Faith Kabata and Donrich Thaldar, 'The Human Genome as the Common Heritage of Mankind', *Frontiers in Genetics* 14 (2023): 1282515.
43 Christiane Nüsslein-Volhard, 'Manipulating the Human Embryo', *USA Today* (2011): 30.
44 Ibid.
45 Ball, *Unnatural*, 167.
46 Ibid., 189.
47 Peter Firchow, 'Science and Conscience in Huxley's "Brave New World"', *Contemporary Literature* 16, no. 3 (1975): 301, 303.

48 D. S. Ferber, '"Miracle in Iowa": Metaphor, Analogy, and Anachronism in the History of Bioethics', *Monash Bioethics Review* 23, no. 3 (2004): 7.
49 George P. Smith II, 'Intimations of Immortality: Clones, Cyrons and the Law', *U.N.S.W. Law Journal* 6 (1983): 121.
50 Walters, 'Cloning, Ectogenesis, and Hybrids: Things to Come?', 116.
51 Philip Ball, 'The Art of Medicine: Unnatural Reactions', *Lancet* 383 (2014): 1964.
52 Andrew Milner, J. R. Burgmann, Rjurik Davidson and Susan Cousin, 'Ice, Fire, Flood: Science Fiction and the Anthropocene', *Thesis Eleven* 131, no. 1 (2015): 13.
53 Fred Schiller (writer), Tony Akins (penciller) and Jim Brozman (inker), 'Factories', *The Terminator* #11 (Chicago: NOW Comics, 1989); Schiller, Akins and Brozman, 'Night Convoy', *The Terminator* #12 (Chicago: NOW Comics, 1989), 1–4, 15.
54 Weber, *At All Costs.*
55 Lois McMaster Bujold, *Ethan of Athos* (New York: Baen Books, 1986).
56 Jinal Dadiya, 'Medical Need and Medicalisation in Funding Assisted Reproduction: A Right to Health Analysis', *Medical Law International* 22, no. 3 (2022): 249.
57 Guy Immega, *Super-Earth Mother: The AI that Engineered a Brave New World* (EDGE-Lite, 2023), Kindle eBook location 98, 107.
58 Ibid., 107.
59 Konrad Szocik, 'Humanity Should Colonise in Order to Survive But Not with Embryo Space Colonization', *International Journal of Astrobiology* 20, no. 4 (2021): 319–22; Matthew R. Edwards, 'Space Ectogenesis: Securing Survival of Humans and Earth Life with Minimal Risks – Reply to Szocik', *International Journal of Astrobiology* 20, no. 4 (2021): 323–6; Evie Kendal, 'Ectogenesis and the Ethics of New Reproductive Technologies for Space Exploration', in *Transhumanism: Entering an Era of Bodyhacking and Radical Human Modification*, Emma Tumilty and Michele Battle-Fisher (eds) (Cham: Springer, 2022), 211–26.
60 Matthew R. Edwards, 'Android Noahs and Embryo Arks: Ectogenesis in Global Catastrophe Survival and Space Colonization', *International Journal of Astrobiology* 20, no. 2 (2021): 150–8; Maurizio Balistreri, 'Human Extinction, Artificial Womb and Intelligent Machines', *International Journal of Philosophy* 37, no. 1 (2023): 11–30.
61 Maurizio Balistreri and Steven Umbrello, 'Should the Colonisation of Space Be Based on Reproduction? Critical Considerations on the Choice of Having a Child in Space', *Journal of Responsible Technology* 11 (2020): 100040; Evie Kendal, 'Desire, Duty, and Discrimination: Is There an Ethical Way to Select Human's for Noah's Ark?' in *Reclaiming Space: Progressive and Multicultural Visions of Space Exploration*, J. S. J. Schwartz, Linda Billings and Erika Nesvold (eds) (Oxford: Oxford University Press, 2023), 289.

62 Garrett Hardin, 'Lifeboat Ethics: The Case against Helping the Poor', *Psychology Today* 8 (1974): 38–43.

63 Larry Niven et al., *The Dragons of Heorot* (London: Gollancz, 1995).

64 Evie Kendal, 'Ectogenesis for Space Exploration', in *eLS* 2 (2021): 1–5.

65 Immega, *Super-Earth Mother*, 653.

66 Ibid., 208.

67 CRISPR is a form of gene editing and stands for clustered regularly interspaced short palindromic repeats.

68 Immega, *Super-Earth Mother*, 217.

69 I. Glenn Cohen, 'The Right Not to Be a Genetic Parent?', *Southern California Law Review* 81 (2007): 1126–7.

70 Ibid., 1149.

71 Terry Kavanagh (writer), Roger Cruz (penciller), Rud LaRosa and Wellington Diaz (inkers), 'Breeding Ground', *X-man,* Volume 1, #-1 (New York: Marvel Comics Group, 1997); Grant Morrison (writer), Andy Kubert (penciller) and Jesse Delperdang (inker), 'Batman in Bethlehem', *Batman*, Volume 1 #666, in *Batman and Son* (Burbank, California: DC Comics, 2007), 181; Scott Lobdell (writer), R. B. Silva (illustrator) and Rob Lean (illustrator). 'Incubation', DC New 52 *Superboy*, volume 1 #1–7 (Burbank, California: DC Comics, 2011).

72 Dion Farquhar, '(M)other Discourses', in *The Gendered Cyborg: A Reader*, Gill Kirkup, Kathryn Woodward and Fiona Hovenden (eds) (London: Routledge, 2000), 211, 213.

73 Farquhar, *The Other Machine*, 32.

74 This point is further discussed in the 'bathtub' thought experiment in Cohen, 'The Right Not to Be a Genetic Parent?' 1125, considered in the next chapter.

75 Rosi Braidotti, 'Mothers, Monsters, and Machines', in *Writing on the Body: Female Embodiment and Feminist Theory*, Katient Conboy, Nadia Medina and Saran Stanbury (eds) (New York: Columbia University Press, 1997), 71.

76 Jeremy Rifkin, 'Evolution's Pregnant Pause: Artificial Wombs', *Los Angeles Times*, 21 January 2002, Accessed 24 January 2024, https://www.latimes.com/archives/la-xpm-2002-jan-21-oe-rifkin21-story.html; *see also,* Jeremy Rifkin, *The Biotech Century: Harnessing the Gene and Remaking the World* (New York: Putnam, 1998), 30.

77 Ibid.

78 Tong, *Feminist Thought*, 79.

79 Braidotti, 'Mothers, Monsters, and Machines', 63.

80 Ruth Colker, *Pregnant Men: Practice, Theory, and the Law* (Bloomington: Indiana University Press, 1994), 143.

81 Raymond, 'Maternal Environments and Ejaculatory Fathers', 65.

82 Steiger, 'Not of Woman Born', 151.

83 Alice Adam, 'Out of the Womb: The Future of the Uterine Metaphor', *Feminist Studies* 19, no. 2 (1993): 275.
84 Marge Piercy, *Woman on the Edge of Time* (New York: Ballantine Books, 1976).
85 Kathy Rudy, 'Ethics, Reproduction, Utopia: Gender and Childbearing in "Woman on the Edge of Time" and "The Left Hand of Darkness"', *NWSA Journal* 9, no. 1 (1997): 31–6.
86 Livingston, 'The Biology of Utopia', 285.
87 Farquhar, *The Other Machine*, 32.
88 Ibid.
89 Ball, *Unnatural*, 181.
90 Vera Brittain, *Halcyon, or the Future of Monogamy* (London: Kegan Paul, Trench, Trubner, 1929).
91 Susan M. Squier, 'Reproducing the Posthuman Body: Ectogenetic Fetus, Surrogate Mother, Pregnant Man', in *Posthuman Bodies*, Judith Halberstam and Ira Livingston (eds) (Bloomington: Indiana University Press, 1995), 118.
92 *The Pod Generation*, [Film] directed by Sophie Barthes (Belgium: Scope Pictures, 2023).
93 Ibid.
94 Ibid.
95 Ibid.
96 Ibid.
97 Ibid.
98 Ibid.
99 Ibid.
100 Helen Sedgwick, *The Growing Season* (London: Harvill Seeker, 2017).
101 Ibid.
102 Lee M. Silver, *Remaking Eden: Cloning, Genetic Engineering and the Future of Humankind?* (London: Phoenix Giant, 1998), 10.
103 Ibid.
104 Aline Ferreira, 'The Sexual Politics of Ectogenesis in the To-day and To-morrow Series', *Interdisciplinary Science Reviews* 34, no. 1 (2009): 32.

4 Bioethics engaging with science fiction

1 An earlier version of this chapter is published as: Evie Kendal, 'Utopian Visions of "Making People": Science Fiction and Debates on Cloning, Ectogenesis, Genetic Engineering, and Genetic Discrimination', in *Biopolitics and Utopia: An Interdisciplinary Reader*, Patricia Stapleton and Andrew Byers (eds.) (New York: Palgrave Macmillan, 2015), 89–117.

2 Tranter, 'The Speculative Jurisdiction', 818.
3 Vint, 'Introduction', 161.
4 Huxley, *Brave New World.*
5 *Gattaca*, [Film] directed by Andrew Niccol (California: Columbia Pictures Corporation, 1997).
6 Shelley, *Frankenstein*, 171.
7 Michel Foucault, *The History of Sexuality: An Introduction Volume I* (New York: Vintage Books, 1990), 139.
8 Ibid.
9 This fits Foucault's model, which states that the *anatomo-politics of the human body* involves 'its disciplining, the optimization of its capabilities, the extortion of its forces, the parallel increase of its usefulness and its docility, its integration into systems of efficient and economic controls'. Ibid.
10 A. R. T. Schuck and C. H. de Vreese, 'Between Risk and Opportunity: News Framing and Its Effects on Public Support for EU Enlargement', *European Journal of Communication* 21, no. 1 (2006): 6.
11 George Y. Bizer, Jeff T. Larsen and Richard E. Petty, 'Exploring the Valence-Framing Effect: Negative Framing Enhances Attitude Strength', *Political Psychology* 32, no. 1 (2011): 65.
12 Perri Klass, 'The Artificial Womb Is Born', *The New York Times* online, 29 September 1996. Accessed 12 November 2014. http://www.nytimes.com/1996/09/29/magazine/the-artificial-womb-is-born.html?
13 Anonymous, 'The Artificial Womb Is Born and the World of the Matrix Begins', *ConsciousNewsMedia* online, 11 July 2013. Accessed 12 November 2014: http://consciousnewsmedia.blogspot.com.au/2013/11/the-artificial-womb-is-born-and-world.html#
14 Mark Lallanilla, 'Human Embryos Created without Egg or Sperm in Controversial Breakthrough', *New York Post*, 15 June 2023. Accessed 15 February 2024. https://nypost.com/2023/06/15/human-embryos-created-without-egg-or-sperm-in-controversial-breakthrough/; F. D. Flam, 'Don't Squander a Key Advance in Fertility Research', *Bloomberg*, 25 June 2023. Accessed 15 February 2024. https://www.bloomberg.com/opinion/articles/2023-06-25/don-t-squander-a-key-advance-in-fertility-research?
15 Elizabeth Rayne, 'Brave New World Is Being Reinvented with Synthetic Embryos – and the Right Reasons', *Syfy*, 1 May 2021. Accessed 15 February 2024. https://www.syfy.com/syfy-wire/brave-new-world-reinvented-with-synthetic-embryos
16 Philip Ball, 'Are Human Embryo Models a Cause for Hope or Alarm?' *The Guardian*, 1 July 2023. Accessed 15 February 2024. https://www.theguardian.com/science/2023/jul/01/are-human-embryo-models-a-cause-for-hope-or-alarm
17 Ibid.

18 Wesley J. Smith, 'About Those "Synthetic Embryos"', *National Review*, 8 August 2022. Accessed 15 February 2024. https://www.nationalreview.com/corner/about-those-synthetic-embryos/
19 Tranter, 'The Speculative Jurisdiction', 826.
20 Ibid., 827.
21 Ibid., 836.
22 Robert J. Favole, 'Artificial Gestation: New Meaning for the Right to Terminate a Pregnancy', *Arizona Law Review* 21 (1979): 760.
23 Bridget M. Fuselier, 'The Wisdom of Solomon: We Cannot Split the Pre-embryo', *Cardozo Journal of Law and Gender* 17 (2010–11): 511.
24 Cohen, 'The Right Not to Be a Genetic Parent?', 1125.
25 Hamilton, 'Traces of the Future', 267.
26 Ibid.
27 Jane Maienschein, 'Part II: What's in a Name: Embryos, Clones, and Stem Cells', *American Journal of Bioethics* 2, no. 1 (2002): 16.
28 Ibid., 17.
29 Christopher Benjamin Menadue, et al., 'An Empirical Revision of the Definition of Science Fiction: It Is All in the Techne...', *SAGE Open* 10, no. 4 (2020): 1–18.
30 Jesse Weiner, et al., 'Introduction: The Modern Prometheus Turns 200', in *Frankenstein and Its Classics: The Modern Prometheus from Antiquity to Science Fiction,* Jesse Weiner, et al. (eds.) (London: Bloomsbury Academic, 2018), 7.
31 Menadue, et al., 'An Empirical Revision', 2.
32 Kate Stanton, 'Sounds Like Science Fiction', *Pursuit*, 27 December 2017. Accessed 19 February 2024. https://pursuit.unimelb.edu.au/articles/sounds-like-science-fiction
33 Ibid.
34 Nicholas Agar, *Liberal Eugenics: In Defence of Human Enhancement* (Malden: Blackwell Publishing, 2004).
35 Nancy C. Jones, 'Scientism or Luddism: Is Informed Ethical Possible?' *American Journal of Bioethics* 4, no. 1 (2004): 18.
36 Chris Mason, 'Making People: Today's Wariness of Reproductive Technologies Stems from Myths, Legends and Hollywood', *Nature* 471, no. 7338 (2011): 297.
37 Ted Peters and Gaymon Bennett, Jr., 'Stem Cell Research and the Claim of the Other in the Human Subject', *Dialog: A Journal of Theology* 43, no. 3 (2004): 185.
38 S. Philip Morgan, et al., 'Brave New Worlds: Philosophy, Politics, and Science in Human Biotechnology', *Population and Development Review* 31, no. 1 (2005): 131.
39 Ronald M. Green, *Babies by Design: The Ethics of Genetic Choice* (New Haven: Yale University Press, 2008).
40 Dena S. Davis, 'From YUCK to WOW and Back Again: A Review Article', *Religious Studies Review* 35, no. 3 (2009): 147.

41 Hilary S. Crew, 'Not So Brave a World: The Representation of Human Cloning in Science Fiction for Young Adults', *The Lion and the Unicorn* 28, no. 2 (2004): 204.
42 Hamilton, 'Traces of the Future', 278.
43 Tranter, 'The Speculative Jurisdiction', 838.
44 Jenny Kitzinger, 'Questioning the Sci-Fi Alibi: A Critique of How "Science Fiction Fears" Are Used to Explain Away Public Concerns about Risk', *Journal of Risk Research* 13, no. 1 (2010): 73–86.
45 Ibid., 74.
46 Ibid.
47 Ibid.
48 Ibid., 77.
49 Rosemary Robins, 'Public and Popular Representations of "Frankenscience"', *Social Studies of Science* 29, no. 2 (1999): 295–301.
50 Anne Murcott, 'Public Beliefs about GM Foods: More on the Makings of a Considered Sociology', *Medical Anthropology Quarterly* 15, no. 1 (2001): 15.
51 Latimer, 'Reproductive Technologies, Fetal Icons, and Genetic Freaks', 325.
52 Sandra Shapshay, 'Lifting the Genetic Veil of Ignorance: Is There Anything Really Unjust about Gattacan Society?' in *Bioethics at the Movies*, Sandra Shapshay (ed.) (Baltimore: John Hopkins University Press, 2009), 88.
53 Samantha Seiple and Todd Seiple, *Mutants, Clones and Killer Corn: Unlocking the Secrets of Biotechnology* (Minneapolis: Lerner Publications Company, 2005).
54 Emma Hughes and Jenny Kitzinger, 'Science Fiction Fears: An Analysis of How People Use Science Fiction in Discussing Risk and Emerging Science and Technology', *Social Contexts and Responses to Risk Network (SCARR)*, Working Paper no. 28, 2008.
55 Ibid.
56 G. Pascal Zachary, 'Ethics for a Very Small World', *Foreign Policy* 137 (2003): 45.
57 Mason, 'Making People', 297.
58 Ibid., 299.
59 Ann Jurecic and Daniel Marchalik, 'From Literature to Medicine: Dr Frankenstein's Bioethical Experiment', *Lancet* 386 (2015): 1223.
60 Kinling Lo, 'China's Gene-Editing "Frankenstein" Jailed for Three Years in Modified Baby Case', *South China Morning Post*, 30 December 2019. Accessed 19 February 2024. https://www.scmp.com/news/china/science/article/3043894/chinas-gene-editing-frankenstein-jailed-3-years-modified-baby
61 Derek So, 'From Goodness to Good Looks: Changing Images of Human Germline Genetic Modification', *Bioethics* 36 (2022): 564.
62 Ibid.
63 Adam J. Gross, 'Dr. Frankenstein, or: How I Learned to Stop Worrying and Love CRISPR-Cas9', *Jurimetrics* 56, no. 4 (2016): 413–47.

64 Ibid., 447.
65 A prime example can be found in Eileen Hunt Botting, '*Frankenstein* and the Question of Children's Rights *After* Human Germline Genetic Modification', in *Reproductive Ethics II*, L. Campo-Engelstein and P. Burcher (eds.) (Cham: Springer, 2018), 9–24.
66 David A. Kirby, 'The New Eugenics in Cinema: Genetic Determinism and Gene Therapy in "GATTACA"', *Science Fiction Studies* 27, no. 2 (2000): 199.
67 David A. Kirby, 'The Devil in Our DNA: A Brief History of Eugenics in Science Fiction Films', *Literature and Medicine* 26, no. 1 (2007): 84.
68 Lee Easton, 'Passing Genes in GATTACA, or Straight Genes for the Queer Guy', in *The Influence of Imagination: Essays on Science Fiction and Fantasy as Agents of Social Change*, Lee Easton and Randy Schroeder (eds.) (Jefferson: McFarland & Company, 2007), 70–1.
69 Shapshay, 'Lifting the Genetic Veil', 88.
70 Curtis A. Kin, 'Coming Soon to the "Genetic Supermarket" Near You', *Stanford Law Review* 48, no. 6 (1996): 1573.
71 Lantos and Janvier, 'The Dilemmas of Artificial Wombs', 83.
72 Silver, 'Remaking Eden', 10.
73 Wolpert, 'The Medawar Lecture 1998', 1256.
74 Sarah Chan, 'More Than Cautionary Tales: The Role of Fiction in Bioethics', [editorial] *Journal of Medical Ethics* 35, no. 7 (2009): 398–9.
75 Chan, 'More Than Cautionary Tales', 398.
76 Chambers, *The Fiction of Bioethics*, 2; Ibid.
77 Hellsten, 'Popular Metaphors of Biosciences', 22.
78 Ibid., 16–17.
79 Maienschein, 'Part II: What's in a Name?', 15.
80 Vint, 'Introduction', 161.
81 Hamilton, 'Traces of the Future', 268–70.
82 Squier, 'Reproducing the Posthuman Body', 113–132; Latimer, 'Reproductive Technologies', 332.
83 Jennifer C. Lahl, 'Caveat Emptor', *American Journal of Bioethics* 4, no. 1 (2004): 20.
84 Nick Bostrom, 'In Defence of Posthuman Dignity', *Bioethics* 19, no. 3 (2005): 206.
85 Chan, 'More Than Cautionary Tales', 398.
86 Gregory E. Pence, *Who's Afraid of Human Cloning?* (Lanham: Rowman and Littlefield Publishers, 1998), 39–40.
87 Lee M. Silver, 'Genetics Goes to Hollywood', *Nature Genetics* 17 (1997): 260.
88 Françoise Baylis and Jason Scott Robert, 'The Inevitability of Genetic Enhancement Technologies', *Bioethics* 18, no. 1 (2004): 19.
89 Ibid., 15.

90 Ken McLeod, 'GATTACA', in *The Influence of Imagination: Essays on Science Fiction and Fantasy as Agents of Social Change*, Lee Easton and Randy Schroeder (eds.) (Jefferson: McFarland & Company, 2007), 176.

91 Howard Brody, 'Literature and Bioethics: Different Approaches?' *Literature and Medicine* 10 (1991): 98.

92 Juan Jorge Michel Fariña, 'A Model for Teaching Bioethics and Human Rights Through Cinema and Popular TV Series: A Methodological Approach', *Counselling Psychology Quarterly* 22, no. 1 (2009): 109.

93 Cartwright, *Moral Spectatorship*, 56.

94 James J. Hughes and John D. Lantos, 'Medical Ethics through the Star Trek Lens', *Literature and Medicine* 20, no. 1 (2001):

95 James J. Hughes and John D. Lantos, 'Medical Ethics through the Star Trek Lens', *Literature and Medicine* 20, no. 1 (2001): 32.

96 Ibid.

97 Biggers, 'IVF and Embryo Transfer', 119.

98 Ibid.

99 Patrick D. Hopkins, 'Bad Copies: How Popular Media Represent Cloning as an Ethical Problem', *The Hastings Center Report* 28, no. 2 (1998): 11.

100 Firchow, 'Science and Conscience in Huxley's "Brave New World"', 300.

101 For example, Rita Arditti notes that science and technology is not 'value-free' but rather 'permeated by the same patriarchal values that dominate every other sphere of influence and power in society'. Rita Arditti, 'Reducing Women to Matter', *Women's Studies International Forum* 8, no. 6 (1985): 577.

102 Martin Thomasson, 'A Very Wise Child – Ectogenesis and the Biological Family', *The Family in the Age of Biotechnology*. Carole Ulanowsky (ed.) (Suffolk: Ipswich Book Co, 1995), 79

103 John Edwards, 'New Conceptions: Biosocial Innovations and the Family', *Journal of Marriage and Family* 53, no. 2 (1991): 358.

104 H. Bruce Franklin, *Future Perfect: American Science Fiction of the Nineteenth Century: An Anthology* (Oxford and New York: Oxford University Press, 1966), 1.

105 Istvan Csicsery-Ronay, Jr., 'The SF of Theory: Baudrillard and Haraway', *Science Fiction Studies* 18, no. 3 (1991): 387; Eugene Thacker, 'SF, Technoscience, Net. art: The Politics of Extrapolation', *Art Journal* 59, no. 3 (2000): 66.

106 Fredric Jameson, 'Progress versus Utopia; or, Can We Imagine the Future?' *Science Fiction Studies* 9, no. 2 (1982): 147.

107 Csicsery-Ronay, Jr., 'The SF of Theory', 387.

108 Hamilton, 'Traces of the Future', 267.

109 Kirby, 'The Devil in Our DNA', 97; Kirby, 'The New Eugenics', 196.

110 Fredric Jameson, *Archaeologies of the Future: The Desire Called Utopia and Other Science Fiction* (London: Verso, 2005), 81.

111 Ursula K. Le Guin, *The Left Hand of Darkness* (New York: Ace Books, 1969).
112 Susan M. Squier, *Liminal Lives: Imagining the Human at the Frontiers of Biomedicine* (Durham: Duke University Press, 2004), 212.
113 Sargent, 'Authority and Utopia: Utopianism in Political Thought', 566.
114 Mulford Q. Sibley, 'Apology for Utopia II: Utopia and Politics', *Journal of Politics* 2, no. 2 (1940): 186.

5 Things to do with (science fiction) stories

1 Nelson, 'Introduction', viii.
2 Catherine Belling, 'The Living Dead: Fiction, Horror, and Bioethics', *Perspectives in Biology and Medicine* 53, no. 3 (2010): 440.
3 Brody, 'Literature and Bioethics', 99.
4 Ibid., 107.
5 Harold Braswell, 'Taking Representation Seriously: Rethinking Bioethics Through Clint Eastwood's *Million Dollar Baby*', *Journal of Medical Humanities* 32 (2011): 77.
6 Brody, 'Literature and Bioethics', 108–9.
7 Ibid., 109.
8 Christina Bieber Lake, *Prophets of the Posthuman: American Fiction, Biotechnology, and the Ethics of Personhood* (Indiana: University of Notre Dame Press, 2013), 33.
9 Eric S. Rabkin, 'Science Fiction and Bioethical Knowledge', in *Bioethics and Biolaw through Literature*, Daniela Carpi (ed.) (Berlin: De Gruyter, 2011), 138, 140.
10 Joan Slonczewski 'An Interview with Joan Slonczewski', in *Posthuman Biopolitics: The Science Fiction of Joan Slonczewski*, Bruce Clarke (ed.) (Cham: Palgrave Macmillan, 2020), 10.
11 Ibid.
12 Belling, 'The Living Dead', 445.
13 Ibid., 446.
14 Ibid., 440–1.
15 Ibid., 449.
16 Kaori Sasaki, 'Bioethics Between Imaginary and Reality: Tracing Science Fiction and Its Shaping of Transplant Medicine Protocols in Japan', *East Asian Science, Technology and Society: An International Journal* 13, no. 1 (2019): 77–99.
17 Ibid., 78.
18 Ibid., 79–80.
19 Ibid., 94.
20 Ibid.
21 Ibid., 95.
22 Ibid.

23 Ibid., 88, 91.
24 Nicola Gavioli, 'Bioethical Issues in Contemporary Brazilian Culture: Euthanasia and Literature', *Luso-Brazilian Review* 54, no. 2 (2017): 131.
25 Ibid., 130.
26 Nelson, 'Introduction', xiv.
27 Belling, 'The Living Dead', 439.
28 Priscilla Wald, 'The Art of Medicine: Cognitive Estrangement, Science Fiction and Medical Ethics', *The Lancet* 371 (2008): 1908.
29 Huxley, *Brave New World.*
30 Zimmerman, 'Technology and the Future of Women', 355.
31 Ibid., 364.
32 Brody, 'Literature and Bioethics', 99.
33 Nelson, 'Introduction', ix.
34 Ibid.
35 Gerald Prince, 'Narrative Analysis and Narratology', *New Literary History* 13, no. 2 (1982): 179.
36 Wolf Schmid, *Narratology: An Introduction*, Alexander Starritt (trans.) (Berlin: Walter de Gruyer, 2010), 2.
37 Prince, 'Narrative Analysis and Narratology', 181.
38 Peter Verstraten, *Film Narratology*, Stefan van der Lecq (trans) (Toronto: University of Toronto Press, 2009), 12; Andrew L. LaFave and Elizabeth A. Mainz, 'Engaging with the *Syuzhet*: A New Methodological Approach to Analyzing and Visualizing Internet Discourse', *Ethnography* 19, no. 2 (2018): 185.
39 Mieke Bal, *Narratology: Introduction to the Theory of Narrative* 3rd edition (Toronto: University of Toronto Press, 2009), 5; Stephen J. Carter, 'The Narratable/in Mieke Bal and Jean Baudrillard', *Critical Survey* 7, no. 3 (1995): 339.
40 Delany, *Starboard Wine*, 153.
41 David Herman, 'Scripts, Sequences, and Stories: Elements of a Postclassical Narratology'. *PMLA* 112, no. 5 (1997): 1048.
42 Verstraten, *Film Narratology*, 12.
43 Ibid., 21–2.
44 David Bordwell, *Poetics of Cinema* (Oxfordshire: Routledge, 2008), 13.
45 Hellsten, 'Popular Metaphors of Biosciences', 16-17.
46 Verstraten, *Film Narratology*, 25.
47 Tilmann Köppe and Tom Kindt, 'Unreliable Narration with a Narrator and without' *Journal of Literary Theory* 5, no. 1 (2011): 87.
48 John C. Stys, 'Documentary Bioethics: Visual Narratives for Generations X and Y', *Journal of Medical Humanities* 27, no. 1 (2006): 58.
49 Lindemann, 'In the Matter of Stories', 94.

50 Henry James, 'The Art of Fiction', in Henry James, *Partial Portraits* (London: Macmillan and Co., Limited, 1899), 375–408.

51 Gérard Genette, *Narrative Discourse: An Essay in Method*, Jane E. Lewin (trans.) (Ithaca: Cornell University Press, 1980), 189. The formulations used here are derived from Tzvetan Todorov, 'Les Catégories du Récit Littéraire [The Categories of Literary Narrative]', Joseph Ketner (trans.), *Papers on Language and Literature* 50, no. 3–4 (2014): 381–424.

52 Dan Shen, 'Stylistics, Narratology, and Point of View: Partiality, Complementarity, and a New Definition', *Style* 57, no. 4 (2023): 415.

53 Ibid.

54 Ibid., 189–90.

55 Sabine Schlickers, 'Focalization, Ocularization and Auricularization in Film and Literature', in *Point of View, Perspective, and Focalization: Modeling Mediation in Narrative*, Peter Hühn et al. (eds.) (Berlin: Walter de Gruyter, 2009), 246, 253.

56 Schmid, *Narratology*, 93.

57 Wayne C. Booth, *The Rhetoric of Fiction*, 2nd edition (Chicago: Chicago University Press, 1983).

58 Schmid, *Narratology*, 27.

59 Ibid., 29.

60 Julia Epstein, 'The Pregnant Imagination, Fetal Rights, and Women's Bodies: A Historical Inquiry', *Yale Journal of Law & the Humanities* 7, no. 1 (2013): 139.

61 Ibid., 140.

62 Ibid.

63 Marion Gymnich, 'Gender and Narratology', *Literature Compass* 10, no. 9 (2013): 708.

64 Pritha Kundu, '"The Doctor's Dilemma" and Bioethics in Literature: An Interdisciplinary Approach', *Janus Head* 16, no. 1 (2018): 128.

65 Lindemann, 'In the Matter of Stories', 95–6.

66 Ibid., 94.

67 Stys, 'Documentary Bioethics', 65.

68 Jémeljan Hakemulder, *The Moral Laboratory: Experiments Examining the Effects of Reading Literature on Social Perception and Moral Self-concept* (Amsterdam: John Benjamins Publishing Company, 2000), 37.

69 Ibid., 7, 13, 16.

70 Gymnich, 'Gender and Narratology', 705.

71 Ibid., 706.

72 Ibid., 705.

73 Susan S. Lanser, 'Toward a Feminist Narratology', *Style* 20, no. 3 (1986): 344.

74 Ibid., 354.

75 Susan S. Lanser, *The Narrative Act: Point of View in Prose Fiction* (New Jersey: Princeton University Press, 1981), 92. She also notes that 'when a heterodiegetic narrator's gender is unmarked', there is usually the assumption they are male and straight. Susan S. Lanser, 'Toward (a Queerer and) More (Feminist) Narratology', in *Narrative Theory Unbound: Queer and Feminist Interventions*, Robyn Warhol and Susan S. Lanser (eds.) (Columbus: Ohio State University Press, 2015), 30.
76 Ibid.
77 Ibid., 93.
78 Irene Sanz Alonso, 'Science Fiction Magnifying Mirrors: Octavia Butler's *Dawn* and the Ethics of Genetic Manipulation', *Proceedings of the 31*st *AEDEAN Conference* (2008): 886.
79 Octavia E. Butler, *Dawn* (London: Headline Publishing Group, 2022), 118.
80 Ibid., 235.
81 Ibid., 67.
82 Butler, *Dawn*, 36.
83 Ibid.
84 Éva Federmayer, 'Octavia Butler's Maternal Cyborgs: The Black Female World of the Xenogenesis Trilogy', *Hungarian Journal of English and American Studies* 6, no. 1 (2000): 107–8.
85 Nancy Jesser, 'Blood, Genes and Gender in Octavia Butler's *Kindred* and *Dawn*', *Extrapolation* 43, no. 1 (2002): 52.
86 Butler, *Dawn*, 281–2.
87 Jihun Yoo, 'Transhumanist Impulse, Utopian Vision, and Reversing Dystopia in Margaret Atwood's *Oryx and Crake* and Octavia E. Butler's *Dawn*', *The Modern Language Review* 114, no. 4 (2019): 664.
88 Ibid., 662.
89 Meghan Hurley-Powell, '"We're Never Trapped by Power": A Plurality of Feminist Resistance in Octavia Butler's Dawn', *Journal of Literature, Culture and Literary Translation* 10, no. 1 (2019): 3.
90 Ibid., 2.
91 Butler, *Dawn*, 283.
92 Hurley-Powell, 'We're Never Trapped by Power', 13.
93 Sanz Alonso, 'Science Fiction Magnifying Mirrors', 886.
94 Ibid., 881. For Joanna Russ, this represents how science fiction can be literature and yet not able to be 'judged by the usual literary criteria'. Joanna Russ, 'Towards an Aesthetic of Science Fiction', *Science Fiction Studies* 2 (1976): 112.
95 Suvin, 'On What Is and Is Not an SF Narration', 45.
96 Yoo, 'Transhumanist Impulse', 679.
97 Ibid., 674.

98 Hurley-Powell, 'We're Never Trapped by Power', 3.

99 Ibid., 4.

100 Ibid., 7.

101 Justin Louis Mann, 'Pessimistic Futurism: Survival and Reproduction in Octavia Butler's *Dawn*', *Feminist Theory* 19, no. 1 (2017): 71.

102 Ibid., 62.

103 Butler, *Dawn*, 181.

104 Ibid.

105 Ibid., 184.

106 Ibid., 215.

107 Ibid., 213–14.

108 Ibid., 215.

109 Ibid., 214.

110 Ibid., 216.

111 Ibid., 201.

112 Ibid., 45.

113 Michele Osherow, 'The Dawn of a New Lilith: Revisionary Mythmaking in Women's Science Fiction', *NWSA Journal* 12, no. 1 (2000): 76.

114 Ibid., 76–7.

115 Butler, *Dawn*, 105.

116 Ibid., 105–6.

117 Ibid., 104.

118 Ibid., 104–5.

119 Ibid., 106.

120 Ibid., 108.

121 Ibid., 172.

122 Sanz Alonso, 'Science Fiction Magnifying Mirrors', 886.

123 Ibid., 887.

124 Sami Abdullah Al-Nuaimi, et al., 'Afrofuturism and Transhumanism: New Insights into the African American Identity in Octavia Butler's *Dawn*', *Pertanika Journal of Social Sciences & Humanities* 29, no. 2 (2021): 980–1.

125 Ibid., 982.

126 Florence Okoye, 'Afrofuturism as Intersectional Transhumanism', presentation at *Techno Resistance and Black Future Festival* (Goldsmiths, London, 2017). Accessed 18 March 2024. https://finokoye.files.wordpress.com/2019/08/af_as_it_presentation.pdf; Nicola Bozzi, 'Report: Techno Resistance and Black Future', *Medium*, 6 June 2017. Accessed 18 March 2024. https://medium.com/schizocities/report-techno-resistance-and-black-futures-9e366b8c7d41

127 Jesser, 'Blood, Genes and Gender', 39.

128 Butler, *Dawn*, 40–41.

129 Of this point, Hoda M. Zaki claims: 'To accept Butler's notion that males are genetically (i.e., inherently) more violent than women is to accept an essentialist view of human nature similar to that of some radical feminists, such as Julia Kristeva and Luce Irigaray'. Hoda M. Zaki, 'Utopia, Dystopia, and Ideology in the Science Fiction of Octavia Butler (Utopie, dystopie et idéologie dans la science-fiction d'Octavia Butler)', *Science Fiction Studies* 17, no. 2 (1990): 242.
130 Nelson, 'Introduction', x.
131 Butler, *Dawn*, 3.
132 Ibid., 101.
133 Ibid.
134 Osherow, 'The Dawn of a New Lilith', 80.
135 Zaki, 'Utopia, Dystopia, and Ideology', 244.
136 Ibid.
137 Ibid., 247.
138 Some of the text provided in this section was originally published open access in Evie Kendal, 'The Use of Free Indirect Discourse in J.R. Ward's *Black Dagger Brotherhood* series', *Colloquy: Text, Theory, Critique* 38 (2019): 20–43.
139 Julie Choi, 'Feminine Authority? Common Sense and the Question of Voice in the Novel', *New Literary History* 27, no. 4 (1996): 655.
140 Butler, *Dawn*, 3.
141 Gertrude Schuelke, "Slipping' in Indirect Discourse', *American Speech* 33, no. 2 (1958): 94.
142 Paul Hernadi, 'Dual Perspective: Free Indirect Discourse and Related Techniques', *Comparative Literature* 24, no. 1 (1972), 36.
143 Butler, *Dawn*, 8.
144 Dorrit Cohn, *Transparent Minds: Narrative Modes for Presenting Consciousness in Fiction* (Princeton: Princeton University Press, 1978), 105.
145 Yael Sharvit, 'The Puzzle of Free Indirect Discourse', *Linguistics and Philosophy* 31 (2008): 354.
146 Butler, *Dawn*, 101.
147 Hernadi, 'Dual Perspective', 41.
148 Stefan Oltean, 'A Survey of the Pragmatic and Referential Functions of Free Indirect Discourse', *Poetics Today* 14, no. 4 (1993): 694.
149 Butler, *Dawn*, 218.
150 Ibid., 232.
151 Peter-Paul Verbeek, 'Materializing Morality: Design Ethics and Technological Mediation', *Science, Technology, & Human Values* 31, no. 3 (2006): 361.
152 Elizabeth Chloe Romanis, Seppe Segers and Ben D. de Jong, 'Value Sensitive Design and the Artificial Placenta', *Journal of Medical Ethics* (2024). DOI: 10.1136/jme-2024-110066.

153 Elizabeth Chloe Romanis and Victoria Adkins, 'Artificial Placentas, Pregnancy Loss and Loss-Sensitive Care', *Journal of Medical Ethics* 50, no. 5 (2024): 299–307.
154 Hanne Aagaard and Elisabeth O. C. Hall, 'Mothers' Experiences of Having a Preterm Infant in the Neonatal Care Unit: A Meta-Synthesis', *Journal of Pediatric Nursing* 23, no. 3 (2008): e31.
155 Evie Kendal, 'Form, Function, Perception, and Reception: Visual Bioethics and the Artificial Womb', *Yale Journal of Biology and Medicine* 95 (2022): 375.
156 Aagaard and Hall, 'Mothers' Experiences', e30.
157 Kendal, 'Form, Function, Perception, and Reception', 376.
158 Federmayer, 'Octavia Butler's Maternal Cyborgs', 113.
159 Immega, *Super-Earth Mother*, 653.
160 Ibid., 208.
161 Ibid., 217.
162 Ibid.
163 *The Pod Generation.*
164 JaneMaree Maher, 'Visibly Pregnant: Toward a Placental Body' *Feminist Review* 72 (2002): 102.
165 JaneMaree Maher, 'A Pregnant Man in the Movies: The Visual Politics of Reproduction', *Continuum: Journal of Media & Cultural Studies* 22, no. 2 (2008), 286.
166 Patricia de Vries, 'The Artificial Womb: Speculative Design Meets the Sociotechnical History of Reproductive Labor', in *Interdisciplinarity in the Scholarly Life Cycle: Learning by Examples in Humanities and Social Science Research*, Karin Bijsterveld and Aagje Swinnen (eds.) (Cham: Palgrave Macmillan, 2023), 238.
167 Ibid., 244.
168 Ibid., 239.
169 Ibid., 240.
170 Ibid., 244.
171 Joyce Nabuurs, et al., 'Crafting the Future of the Artificial Womb – Speculative Design as a Tool for Public Engagement with Emerging Technologies', *Futures* 151 (2023): 103184.
172 Tess Johnson and Elizabeth Chloe Romanis, 'The Relationship between Speculation and Translation in Bioethics: Methods and Methodologies', *Monash Bioethics Review* 41, Suppl 1 (2023): S2.
173 Ibid., S3.
174 Gunn, 'How America's Leading Science Fiction Authors Are Shaping Your Future'.
175 Johnson and Romanis, 'The Relationship between Speculation and Translation in Bioethics', S6.
176 Ibid., S16.
177 Latimer, 'Reproductive Technologies, Fetal Icons, and Genetic Freaks', 323.

178 Ibid.

179 Mason, 'Making People', 299.

180 Eric Racine et al., 'The Value and Pitfalls of Speculation about Science and Technology in Bioethics: The Case of Cognitive Enhancement', *Medicine, Health Care and Philosophy* 17, no. 3 (2014): 326–7.

181 Ibid., 327.

182 Ibid.

183 Sarah Langford, 'An End to Abortion? A Feminist Critique of the "Ectogenetic Solution" to Abortion', *Women's Studies International Forum* 31 (2008): 268.

184 Farquhar, *The Other Machine*, 191.

185 Belling, 'The Living Dead', 449.

Conclusion

1 Valentina Adami, 'Women's Reproductive Rights: A Literary Perspective', *Polemos: Journal of Law, Literature and Culture* 6, no. 1 (2012): 114.

2 Rudy, 'Ethics, Reproduction, Utopia', 26.

3 Laura Briggs and Jodi I. Kelber-Kaye, '"There Is No Unauthorized Breeding in Jurassic Park": Gender and the Uses of Genetics', *NWSA Journal* 12, no. 3 (2000): 95,

4 Ruth Levitas, *Utopia as Method: The Imaginary Reconstruction of Society*. Basingstoke: Palgrave Macmillan, 2013, 111.

5 Severance theory permits pregnancy termination on the grounds of promoting women's bodily autonomy. The associated death of the foetus is only ethically tolerated if it can be viewed as an unfortunate side effect of pregnant women exerting their rights in this way and not as the intended goal of abortion. As such, severance theory relies on the so-called 'doctrine of double effect'.

6 Cannold, 'Women, Ectogenesis and Ethical Theory', 57.

7 Segers, 'The Path to Ectogenesis', 59.

8 Gabriela Arguedas-Ramírez and Danielle M. Wenner, 'Reproductive Justice Beyond Borders: Global Feminist Solidarity in the Post-*Roe* Era', *Journal of Law, Medicine & Ethics* 51 (2023): 606–11.

9 Gisela Zaremberg, Constanza Tabbush and Elisabeth Jay Friedman, 'Feminism(s) and Anti-gender Backlash: Lessons from Latin America', *International Feminist Journal of Politics* 23, no. 4 (2021): 527.

10 Guilia Cavaliere, 'Gestation, Equality and Freedom: Ectogenesis as a Political Perspective', *Journal of Medical Ethics* 46 (2020): 78–9.

11 *Ibid*, 78.

12 Jeffery Hall Dobken discusses this issue in 'Physician-Assisted Suicide (PAS)/ Physician-Assisted Death (PAD): The Rise of Lifeboat Ethics', *Journal of American Physicians and Surgeons* 23, no. 4: (2018): 121–4.

13 Chloe Romanis, 'Equality-Enhancing Potential of Novel Forms of Assisted Gestation: Perspectives of Reproductive Rights Advocates', *Bioethics* 37 (2023): 637–46.

14 Alexandra Krendel and Mike Ryder, 'Role of Science Fiction in Conceptualising the Reproductive Future: A Linguistic and Literary Perspective', *Medical Humanities* (2025). DOI: 10.1136/medhum-2024-013207. These authors conducted an empirical study looking at the frequency with which members of the public invoked science-fictional references when commenting on a 2022 viral video showing a fake artificial womb facility. While the person responsible for the 'Ectolife' video claims it was only intended to demonstrate a concept for a future company, many regard the video as a deliberate hoax.

Bibliography

Aagaard, Hanne, and Elisabeth O. C. Hall. 'Mothers' Experiences of Having a Preterm Infant in the Neonatal Care Unit: A Meta-Synthesis'. *Journal of Pediatric Nursing* 23, no. 3 (2008): e26–e36.

Abdullah Al-Nuaimi, Sami, Zainor Izat Zainal, Mohammad Ewan Awang and Noritah Omar. 'Afrofuturism and Transhumanism: New Insights into the African American Identity in Octavia Butler's *Dawn*'. *Pertanika Journal of Social Sciences & Humanities* 29, no. 2 (2021): 977–92.

Adam, Alice. 'Out of the Womb: The Future of the Uterine Metaphor'. *Feminist Studies* 19, no. 2 (1993): 269–89.

Adami, Valentina. 'Between Bioethics and Literature: Representations of (Post) human Identities in Margaret Atwood's *Oryx and Crake* and *The Year of the Flood*'. *Polemos: Journal of Law, Literature and Culture* 6, no. 2 (2012): 249–61.

Adami, Valentina. 'Women's Reproductive Rights: A Literary Perspective'. *Polemos: Journal of Law, Literature and Culture* 6, no. 1 (2012): 101–23.

Adami, Valentina. *Bioethics Through Literature: Margaret Atwood's Cautionary Tales*. Trier: Wissenschaftlicher Verlag Trier, 2011.

Ahmed, Sara. 'The Performativity of Disgust', in *The Cultural Politics of Emotion*, 82–100. London: Routledge, 2004.

Agar, Nicholas. *Liberal Eugenics: In Defence of Human Enhancement*. Malden: Blackwell Publishing, 2004.

Alghrani, Amed, and Margaret Brazier. 'What Is It? Whose It? Re-positioning the Fetus in the Context of Research?' *Cambridge Law Journal* 70, no. 1 (2011): 51–82.

AlJahsh, Muhammad Ahmad Ibrahim. 'Science and Islamic Ethics: Navigating Artificial Womb Technology Through Quranic Principles'. *Heliyon* 10 (2024): e36793.

American Congress of Obstetricians and Gynecologists (ACOG). 'Committee Opinion: Committee on Ethics. Preembryo Research: History, Scientific Background, and Ethical Considerations'. *International Journal of Gynaecology and Obstetrics* 45 (1994): 291–301.

Anker, Suzanne, and Sarah Franklin. 'Specimens as Spectacles: Reframing Fetal Remains'. *Social Texts* 29, no. 1 (2011): 103–25.

Anonymous. 'Without Gasping for Air Safely in the Artificial Womb'. *TU/e News and Events*, 7 April 2022. Accessed 22 January 2024. https://www.tue.nl/en/storage/biomedische-technologie/de-faculteit/news-and-events/news-overview/07-04-2022-without-gasping-for-air-safely-in-the-artificial-womb

Anonymous. 'In Vitro: Space Above and Beyond', wiki, 11 July 2017. Accessed 5 February 2024. https://spaceaboveandbeyond.fandom.com/wiki/In_Vitro

Anonymous. 'The Artificial Womb Is Born and the World of the Matrix Begins', *ConsciousNewsMedia* online, 11 July 2013. Accessed 12 November 2014. http://consciousnewsmedia.blogspot.com.au/2013/11/the-artific ial-womb-is-born-and-world.html#

Arditti, Rita. 'Reducing Women to Matter'. *Women's Studies International Forum* 8, no. 6 (1985): 577–82.

Arens, Jutta, Mark Schoberer, Anne Lohr, Thorsten Orlikowsky, Matthias Seehase, Reint K. Jellema, Jennifer J. Collins, Boris W. Kramer, Thomas Schmitz-Rode and Ulrich Steinseifer. 'NeonatOx: A Pumpless Extracorporeal Lung Support for Premature Neonates'. *Artificial Organs* 35, no. 11 (2011): 997–1001.

Arguedas-Ramírez, Gabriela, and Danielle M. Wenner. 'Reproductive Justice Beyond Borders: Global Feminist Solidarity in the Post-*Roe* Era'. *Journal of Law, Medicine & Ethics*, 51 (2023): 606–11.

Baehr, Amy R. 'Liberal Feminism', in *The Stanford Encyclopedia of Philosophy*. Edward N. Zalta (ed.), 2021. Accessed 31 January 2025. https://plato.stanford.edu/archives/spr2021/entries/feminism-liberal

Baker, Jeffery P. 'The Incubator and the Medical Discovery of the Premature Infant'. *Journal of Perinatalogy* 5 (2000): 321–8.

Baker, Jeffery P. 'The Incubator Controversy: Pediatricians and the Origins of Premature Infant Technology in the United States, 1890 to 1910'. *Pediatrics* 87, no. 5 (1991): 654–62.

Bal, Mieke. *Narratology: Introduction to the Theory of Narrative* 3rd edition. Toronto: University of Toronto Press, 2009.

Ball, Philip. 'Are Human Embryo Models a Cause for Hope or Alarm?' *The Guardian*, 1 July 2023. Accessed 15 February 2024. https://www.theguardian.com/science/2023/jul/01/are-human-embryo-models-a-cause-for-hope-or-alarm

Ball, Philip. 'The Art of Medicine: Unnatural Reactions'. *The Lancet*, 383 (2014): 1964–5.

Ball, Philip. *Unnatural: The Heretical Idea of Making People*. London: The Bodley Head, 2011.

Balistreri, Maurizio. 'Human Extinction, Artificial Womb and Intelligent Machines'. *International Journal of Philosophy*, 37, no. 1 (2023): 11–30.

Balistreri, Maurizio, and Steven Umbrello. 'Should the Colonisation of Space Be Based on Reproduction? Critical Considerations on the Choice of Having a Child in Space'. *Journal of Responsible Technology* 11 (2020): 100040.

Baylis, Françoise, and Jason Scott Robert. 'The Inevitability of Genetic Enhancement Technologies'. *Bioethics* 18, no. 1 (2004): 1–26.

Bayne, Tim, and Avery Kolers. 'Towards a Pluralist Account of Parenthood'. *Bioethics* 17, no. 3 (2003): 221–42.

Belling, Catherine. 'The Living Dead: Fiction, Horror, and Bioethics'. *Perspectives in Biology and Medicine* 53, no. 3 (2010): 439–51.

Benagiano, Giuseppe, Sabina Carrara and Valentina Filippi. 'Robert G Edwards and the Roman Catholic Church'. *Reproductive Biomedicine Online* 22 (2011): 665–72.

Berkeley, George. *The Works of George Berkeley, Bishop of Cloyne*, Volume 2. A. A. Luce and T. E. Jessop (eds). London: Nelson, 1948.

Biggers, John D. 'IVF and Embryo Transfer: Historical Origin and Development'. *Reproductive Biomedicine Online* 25, no. 2 (2012): 118–27.

Binns, Corey. 'The Shark Factory: An Artificial Uterus Gives an Endangered Species a Shot at Survival'. *Popular Science* 275, no. 1 (2009): 34.

Bizer, George Y., Jeff T. Larsen and Richard E. Petty. 'Exploring the Valence-Framing Effect: Negative Framing Enhances Attitude Strength'. *Political Psychology* 32, no. 1 (2011): 59–80.

Booth, Wayne C. *The Rhetoric of Fiction*, 2nd edition. Chicago: Chicago University Press, 1983.

Bordwell, David. *Poetics of Cinema*. Oxfordshire: Routledge, 2008.

Bostrom, Nick. 'A History of Transhumanist Thought'. *Journal of Evolution & Technology* 14, no. 1 (2005): 1–25.

Bostrom, Nick. 'In Defence of Posthuman Dignity'. *Bioethics* 19, no. 3 (2005): 202–14.

Botting, Eileen Hunt. '*Frankenstein* and the Question of Children's Rights *After* Human Germline Genetic Modification', in *Reproductive Ethics II*. L. Campo-Engelstein and P. Burcher (eds.), 9–24. Cham: Springer, 2018.

Bould, Mark. '*Critical Theory and Science Fiction*, Carl Freedman. Hanover: Wesleyan University Press/University Press of New England, 2000 [review]'. *Historical Materialism* 10, no. 4 (2002): 297–305.

Bozzi, Nicola. 'Report: Techno Resistance and Black Future'. *Medium*, 6 June 2017. Accessed 18 March 2024. https://medium.com/schizocities/report-techno-resistance-and-black-futures-9e366b8c7d41

Braidotti, Rosi. 'Mothers, Monsters, and Machines', in *Writing on the Body: Female Embodiment and Feminist Theory*. Katient Conboy, Nadia Medina and Saran Stanbury (eds), 57–79. New York: Columbia University Press, 1997.

Braswell, Harold. 'Taking Representation Seriously: Rethinking Bioethics Through Clint Eastwood's *Million Dollar Baby*'. *Journal of Medical Humanities* 32 (2011): 77–87.

Briggs, Laura, and Jodi I. Kelber-Kaye. '"There Is No Unauthorized Breeding in Jurassic Park": Gender and the Uses of Genetics'. *NWSA Journal* 12, no. 3 (2000): 92–113.

Brittain, Vera. *Halcyon, or The Future of Monogamy*. London: Kegan Paul, Trench, Trubner, 1929.

Brody, Howard. 'Literature and Bioethics: Different Approaches?' *Literature and Medicine* 10 (1991): 98–110.

Brown, Benjamin Patterson, and Katie Watson. 'No Substitute: The False Promise of Artificial Womb Technology as an Alternative to Abortion'. *American Journal of Bioethics* 23, no. 5 (2023): 87–9.

Browne, Tamara Kayali, Evie Kendal and Tiia Sudenkaarne. 'Feminist Concerns about Artificial Womb Technology'. *American Journal of Bioethics* 23, no. 5 (2023): 97–9.

Bujold, Lois McMaster. *Ethan of Athos*. New York: Baen Books, 1986.

Bujold, Lois McMaster. *Shards of Honor*. New York: Baen Books, 1986.

Bulletti, Carlo, Antonio Palagiano, Caterina Pace, Angelica Cerni, Andrea Borini and Dominique de Ziegler. 'The Artificial Womb'. *Annals of the New York Academy of Science* 1221 (2011): 124–8.

Buran, Sümeyra. 'Being an Artificial Womb Machine-Human', in *Technologies of Feminist Speculative Fiction: Gender, Artificial Life, and the Politics of Reproduction*, Sherryl Vint and Sümeyra Buran (eds), 45–68. Cham: Palgrave, 2022.

Butler, Octavia E. *Dawn*. London: Headline Publishing Group, 2022.

Callahan, Joan C., and James W. Knight. 'Women, Fetuses, Medicine, and the Law', in *Feminist Perspectives in Medical Ethics*. Helen Bequaert Holmes and Laura M. Purdy (eds.), 224–239. Bloomington: Indiana University Press, 1992.

Cannold, Leslie. 'Women, Ectogenesis and Ethical Theory'. *Journal of Applied Philosophy* 12, no. 1 (1995): 55–64.

Carroll, Noël. 'The Wheel of Virtue: Art, Literature, and Moral Knowledge'. *Journal of Aesthetics and Art Criticism* 60, no. 1 (2002): 3–26.

Carroll, Noël. *The Philosophy of Horror: Or, Paradoxes of the Heart*. New York: Routledge, 1990.

Carter, Stephen J. 'The Narratable/in Mieke Bal and Jean Baudrillard'. *Critical Survey* 7, no. 3 (1995): 339–44.

Cartwright, Lisa. *Moral Spectatorship: Technologies of Voice and Affect in Postwar Representations of the Child*. Durham: Duke University Press, 2008.

Case, Mary Anne. 'Feminist Fundamentalism as an Individual and Constitutional Commitment'. *American University Journal of Gender, Social Policy and the Law* 9, no. 2 (2011): 549–76.

Cavaliere, Guilia. 'Gestation, Equality and Freedom: Ectogenesis as a Political Perspective'. *Journal of Medical Ethics* 46 (2020): 76–82.

Chambers, Clare. 'Introduction: A Feminist Liberalism', in *Freedom and Equality: Essays on Liberalism and Feminism*. 1–16. Oxford, Oxford University Press, 2024.

Chambers, Tod. *The Fiction of Bioethics: Cases as Literary Texts*. New York: Routledge, 1999.

Chan, Sarah. 'More Than Cautionary Tales: The Role of Fiction in Bioethics', [editorial]. *Journal of Medical Ethics* 35, no. 7 (2009): 398–9.

Chandler, Daniel. 'Technological or Media Determinism' (1995). Accessed 8 February 2017. http://www.aber.ac.uk/media/Documents/tecdet/tdet01.html

Chavatte-Palmer, P., R. Lévy and P. Boileau. 'Une Reproduction Sans Utérus? État des Lieux de L'ectogenèse [Reproduction without a Uterus? State of the Art of Ectogenesis]'. *Gynécologie Obstétrique and Fertilité* 40, no. 11 (2012): 695–7.

Cheney, Matthew. 'Science Fiction and Difference: *An Introduction to* Starboard Wine', in Samuel R. Delany *Starboard Wine: More Notes on the Language of Science Fiction*. xxi–xxxv. Middleton, Connecticut: Wesleyan University Press, 2012.

Childress, James F. 'Case Narratives and Moral Perspectives: An Appreciative Response to Chambers'. *American Journal of Bioethics* 1, no. 1 (2001): 57–9.

Choi, Julie. 'Feminine Authority? Common Sense and the Question of Voice in the Novel'. *New Literary History* 27, no. 4 (1996): 641–62.

Clayton, Jay. 'The Ridicule of Time: Science Fiction, Bioethics, and the Posthuman'. *American Literary History* 25, no. 2 (2013): 317–43.

Clouser, K. Danner. 'Philosophy, Literature, and Ethics: Let the Engagement Begin'. *Journal of Medicine and Philosophy* 21 (1996): 321–40.

Cohen, I. Glenn. 'The Right Not to Be a Genetic Parent?' *Southern California Law Review* 81 (2007): 1115–96.

Cohn, Dorrit. *Transparent Minds: Narrative Modes for Presenting Consciousness in Fiction*. Princeton: Princeton University Press, 1978.

Colker, Ruth. *Pregnant Men: Practice, Theory, and the Law*. Bloomington: Indiana University Press, 1994.

Conscious News Media. 'The Artificial Womb Is Born and the World of the Matrix Begins'. *ConsciousNewsMedia* online, 11 July 2013. Accessed 12 November 2014. http://consciousnewsmedia.blogspot.com.au/2013/11/the-artificial-womb-is-born-and-world.html#

Cordeiro, James J. 'On the Permissibility of Elective Ectogestation'. *American Journal of Bioethics* 23, no. 5 (2023): 116–18.

Corea, Genoveffa. 'How the New Reproductive Technologies Could be Used to Apply the Brothel Model of Social Control Over Women'. *Women's Studies International Forum* 8, no. 4 (1985): 299–305.

Corea, Genoveffa. *The Mother Machine: Reproductive Technologies from Artificial Insemination to Artificial Wombs*. New York: Harper & Row, 1985.

Crew, Hilary S. 'Not So Brave a World: The Representation of Human Cloning in Science Fiction for Young Adults'. *The Lion and the Unicorn* 28, no. 2 (2004): 203–21.

Csicsery-Ronay, Jr., Istvan. *The Seven Beauties of Science Fiction*. Connecticut: Wesleyan University Press, 2008.

Csicsery-Ronay, Jr., Istvan. 'The SF of Theory: Baudrillard and Haraway'. *Science Fiction Studies* 18, no. 3 (1991): 387–404.

Dadiya, Jinal. 'Medical Need and Medicalisation in Funding Assisted Reproduction: A Right to Health Analysis'. *Medical Law International* 22, no. 3 (2022): 249–74.

Daniels, Cynthia R. 'Fathers, Mothers, and Fetal Harm: Rethinking Gender Difference and Reproductive Responsibility', in *Fetal Subjects, Feminist Positions*. Lynn M. Morgan and Meredith W. Michaels (eds), 83–98. Philadelphia: University of Pennsylvania Press, 1999.

Davis, Dena S. 'From YUCK to WOW and Back Again: A Review Article'. *Religious Studies Review* 35, no. 3 (2009): 24–7.

Davis, Nicola. 'Artificial Womb: Dutch Researchers Given €2.9m to Develop Prototype'. *The Guardian*, 8 October 2019. Accessed 4 October 2021. https://www.theguardian.

com/society/2019/oct/08/artificial-womb-dutch-researchers-given-29m-to-develop-prototype

De Beauvoir, Simone. *The Second Sex*, Constance Borde and Sheila Malovany-Chevallier (trans). London: Vintage Books, 2010.

De Bie, Felix, Sarah D. Kim, Sourav K. Bose, Pamela Nathanson, Emily A. Partridge, Alan W. Flake and Chris Feudtner. 'Ethics Considerations Regarding Artificial Womb Technology for the Fetonate', *American Journal of Bioethics* 23, no. 5 (2023): 67–78.

De Proost, Lien, and Geertjan Zuijdwegt. 'Lost in Gestation: On Fetonates, Perinates, and Gestatelings'. *American Journal of Bioethics* 23, no. 5 (2023): 108–10.

De Vries, Patricia. 'The Artificial Womb: Speculative Design Meets the Sociotechnical History of Reproductive Labor', in *Interdisciplinarity in the Scholarly Life Cycle: Learning by Examples in Humanities and Social Science Research*. Karin Bijsterveld and Aagje Swinnen (eds), 237–51. Cham: Palgrave Macmillan, 2023.

Delany, Samuel R. *Starboard Wine: More Notes on the Language of Science Fiction*. Middleton, Connecticut: Wesleyan University Press, 2012.

Descartes, René. *The Philosophical Writings of Descartes, Volume III: The Correspondence*, John Cottingham et al. (trans). Cambridge: Cambridge University Press, 1991.

DiGregorio, Sarah. 'Artificial Wombs Aren't a Sci-Fi Horror Story'. *Slate*, 30 January 2020. Accessed 22 January 2024. https://slate.com/technology/2020/01/artificial-wombs-science-fiction-pregnancy-premature.html

Dobken, Jeffery Hall. 'Physician-Assisted Suicide (PAS)/Physician-Assisted Death (PAD): The Rise of Lifeboat Ethics'. *Journal of American Physicians and Surgeons* 23, no. 4: (2018): 121–4.

Dubey, Anil K. *Infertility: Diagnosis, Management, & IVF*. New Delhi: Jaypee Brothers Medical Publishers, 2012.

Duden, Barbara. *The Woman Beneath the Skin: A Doctor's Patients in Eighteenth-Century Germany*. Thomas Dunlap (trans). Cambridge: Harvard University Press, 1991.

Dworkin, Andrea. *Right-Wing Women*. New York: Coward-McCann, 1983.

Dworkin, Ronald. *Life's Dominion: An Argument About Abortion, Euthanasia and Individual Freedom*. London: Harper Collins, 1993.

Easton, Lee. 'Passing Genes in GATTACA, or Straight Genes for the Queer Guy', in *The Influence of Imagination: Essays on Science Fiction and Fantasy as Agents of Social Change*. Lee Easton and Randy Schroeder (eds), 70–82. Jefferson: McFarland & Company, 2007.

Edwards, John. 'New Conceptions: Biosocial Innovations and the Family'. *Journal of Marriage and Family* 53, no. 2 (1991): 349–60.

Edwards, Matthew R. 'Space Ectogenesis: Securing Survival of Humans and Earth Life with Minimal Risks – Reply to Szocik'. *International Journal of Astrobiology* 20, no. 4 (2021): 323–6.

Edwards, Matthew R. 'Android Noahs and Embryo Arks: Ectogenesis in Global Catastrophe Survival and Space Colonization'. *International Journal of Astrobiology* 20, no. 2 (2021): 150–8.

Edwards, Robert. *Life Before Birth: Reflections on the Embryo Debate.* London: Hutchinson, 1989.

Epstein, Julia. 'The Pregnant Imagination, Fetal Rights, and Women's Bodies: A Historical Inquiry'. *Yale Journal of Law & the Humanities* 7, no. 1 (2013): 139–62.

Esquerda, Montserrat, David Lorenzo and Margarita Bofarull. 'Beyond the Domains: What Would Be the Fundamental Ethical Questions in the Development of the Artificial Womb'. *American Journal of Bioethics* 23, no. 5 (2023): 125–7.

Fariña, Juan Jorge Michel. 'A Model for Teaching Bioethics and Human Rights Through Cinema and Popular TV Series: A Methodological Approach'. *Counselling Psychology Quarterly* 22, no. 1 (2009): 105–17.

Farquhar, Dion. '(M)other Discourses', in *The Gendered Cyborg: A Reader*. Gill Kirkup, Kathryn Woodward and Fiona Hovenden (eds), 209–20. London: Routledge, 2000.

Farquhar, Dion. *The Other Machine: Discourse and Reproductive Technologies.* New York: Routledge, 1996.

Favole, Robert J. 'Artificial Gestation: New Meaning for the Right to Terminate a Pregnancy'. *Arizona Law Review* 21 (1979): 755–76.

Federmayer, Éva. 'Octavia Butler's Maternal Cyborgs: The Black Female World of the Xenogenesis Trilogy'. *Hungarian Journal of English and American Studies* 6, no. 1 (2000): 103–18.

Ferber, D. S. '"Miracle in Iowa": Metaphor, Analogy, and Anachronism in the History of Bioethics'. *Monash Bioethics Review* 23, no. 3 (2004): 6–15.

Ferreira, Aline. 'The Sexual Politics of Ectogenesis in the To-day and To-morrow Series'. *Interdisciplinary Science Reviews* 34, no. 1 (2009): 32–55.

Firchow, Peter. 'Science and Conscience in Huxley's "Brave New World"'. *Contemporary Literature* 16, no. 3 (1975): 301–16.

Firestone, Shulamith. *The Dialectic of Sex: The Case for Feminist Revolution.* New York: William Morrow and Company, 1970.

Fitting, Peter. 'Utopia, Dystopia and Science Fiction', in *The Cambridge Companion to Utopian Literature*. Gregory Claeys (ed.), 135–53. Cambridge: Cambridge University Press, 2010.

Flam. F. D. 'Don't Squander a Key Advance in Fertility Research'. *Bloomberg*, 25 June 2023. Accessed 15 February 2024. https://www.bloomberg.com/opinion/articles/2023-06-25/don-t-squander-a-key-advance-in-fertility-research?

Fleck, Leonard Michael. 'Abortion, Artificial Wombs, and the "No Difference" Argument'. *American Journal of Bioethics* 23, no. 5 (2023): 94–7.

Forde, Braxton, Marc Oria, Kristin Lampe, Samuel Martin and Jose L. Peiro. 'Creation of a Novel Synthetic Amniotic Fluid for Use in Fetal Therapy with In-vitro Testing on Human Amniotic Membranes'. *American Journal of Obstetrics and Gynecology MFM* 5, no. 9 (2023): 101055.

Foucault, Michel. *The History of Sexuality Volume I: An Introduction*. New York: Vintage Books, 1990.

Franklin, H. Bruce. *Future Perfect: American Science Fiction of the Nineteenth Century: An Anthology*. Oxford and New York: Oxford University Press, 1966.

Freedman, Carl. *Critical Theory and Science Fiction*. Middletown: Wesleyan University Press, 2013.

Fringe, 'The Same Old Story'. Directed by Paul Edwards, written by Jeff Pinkner, J. J. Abrams, Alex Kurtzman and Roberto Orci. Santa Monica: Bad Robot, 16 September 2008.

Frye, Northrop. *On Education*. Ontario: Fitzhenry & Whiteside, 1988.

Frye, Northrop. 'Varieties of Literary Utopia'. *Daedalus* 94, no. 2 (1965): 323–47.

Fuselier, Bridget M. 'The Wisdom of Solomon: We Cannot Split the Pre-Embryo'. *Cardozo Journal of Law and Gender* 17 (2010–11): 507–26.

Garvey, Brian. 'Review: The Utopian Imagination'. *Science Fiction Studies* 15, no. 2 (1988): 244–6.

Gattaca. [Film] Directed by Andrew Niccol. California: Columbia Pictures Corporation, 1997.

Gavina, Tessa, Chris Gastmans and Alice Cavolo. 'Artificial Wombs or Artificial Feminism: What Is Wrong with Being Pregnant?' *American Journal of Bioethics* 23, no. 5 (2023): 104–6.

Gavioli, Nicola. 'Bioethical Issues in Contemporary Brazilian Culture: Euthanasia and Literature'. *Luso-Brazilian Review* 54, no. 2 (2017): 129–51.

Genette, Gérard. 'The Prefactorial Situation of Communication', in *Paratexts: Thresholds of Interpretation*. Cambridge: Cambridge University Press, 2009, 161–95.

Genette, Gérard, *Narrative Discourse: An Essay in Method*, Jane E. Lewin (trans.) Ithaca: Cornell University Press, 1980.

Glock, Hans-Johann (ed.). *A Wittgenstein Dictionary*. *Blackwell Reference Online*, 1996. DOI: 10.1111/b.9780631185376.1996.x

Grant, Edward R. 'The Short-Lived Verdict in *Le Page v Center for Reproductive Medicine*: Why "Personhood" Matters in the Regulation of Assisted Reproductive Technologies'. *Medical Law Review* 32 (2024): 399–409.

Green, Ronald M. *Babies by Design: The Ethics of Genetic Choice*. New Haven: Yale University Press, 2008.

Gross, Adam J. 'Dr. Frankenstein, Or: How I Learned to Stop Worrying and Love CRISPR-Cas9'. *Jurimetrics* 56, no. 4 (2016): 413–47.

Grove, Andy. *Only the Paranoid Survive: How to Exploit the Crisis Points that Challenge Every Company*. New York: Doubleday, 1996.

Gulino, Matteo, Pasquale Ricci and Gianluca Montanari Vergallo. 'Artificial Womb on Maternal Request and without the Father's Consent: Ethical Perspectives Through a Principlist Approach'. *American Journal of Bioethics* 23, no. 5 (2023): 121–3.

Gunn, Eileen. 'How America's Leading Science Fiction Authors Are Shaping Your Future'. *Smithsonian* magazine, May 2014. Accessed 22 January 2024. https://www.

smithsonianmag.com/arts-culture/how-americas-leading-science-fiction-authors-are-shaping-your-future-180951169/

Gymnich, Marion. 'Gender and Narratology'. *Literature Compass* 10, no. 9 (2013): 705–15.

Hailu, Fekade Getachew, Getnet Tesfaye Yihunie, Ahmed Amdihun Essa and Walelign Kindie Tsega. 'Advanced Abdominal Pregnancy, with Live Fetus and Severe Preeclampsia, Case Report'. *BMC Pregnancy and Childbirth* 17 (2017): 243.

Hakemulder, Jémeljan. *The Moral Laboratory: Experiments Examining the Effects of Reading Literature on Social Perception and Moral Self-concept*. Amsterdam: John Benjamins Publishing Company, 2000.

Haldane, J. B. S. *Daedalus: or, Science and the Future: A Paper Read to the Heretics, Cambridge, on February 4th, 1923*. London: Kegan Paul, Trench, Trubner, 1924.

Hamilton, Sheryl N. 'Traces of the Future: Biotechnology, Science Fiction, and the Media'. *Science Fiction Studies* 30, no. 2 (2003): 267–82.

Hardin, Garrett. 'Lifeboat Ethics: The Case Against Helping the Poor'. *Psychology Today* 8 (1974): 38–43.

Haynes, Roslynn. 'From Alchemy to Artificial Intelligence: Stereotypes of the Scientist in Western Literature'. *Public Understanding of Science* 12, no. 3 (2003): 243–53.

Hellsten, Iina. 'Popular Metaphors of Biosciences: Bridges Over Time?' *Configurations* 16, no. 1 (2008): 11–32.

Hernadi, Paul. 'Dual Perspective: Free Indirect Discourse and Related Techniques'. *Comparative Literature* 24, no. 1 (1972): 32–43.

Hendricks, Jennifer S. 'Not of Woman Born: A Scientific Fantasy/'. *Case Western Reserve Law Review* 62 (2012): 1–47.

Heriot, M. Jean. 'Fetal Rights versus the Female Body: Contested Domains'. *Medical Anthropology Quarterly* 10, no. 2 (1996): 176–94.

Herman, David. 'Scripts, Sequences, and Stories: Elements of a Postclassical Narratology'. *PMLA* 112, no. 5 (1997): 1046–59.

Holmes, John, and Laura Hosford. 'Artificial Womb Technology, Catholic Health Care, and Social Justice'. *American Journal of Bioethics* 23, no. 5 (2023): 123–5.

Hopkins, Patrick D. 'Bad Copies: How Popular Media Represent Cloning as an Ethical Problem'. *The Hastings Center Report* 28, no. 2 (1998): 6–13.

Horn, Claire. 'Artificial Wombs, Frozen Embryos, and Parenthood: Will Ectogenesis Redistribute Gendered Responsibility for Gestation?' *Feminist Legal Studies* 30 (2022): 51–72.

Horn, Claire. 'A History of Gestation Outside the Body'. *Wellcome Collection*, 30 November 2021. Accessed 31 January 2025. https://wellcomecollection.org/stories/a-history-of-gestation-outside-the-body

Horn, Claire. 'Ectogenesis Is for Feminists: Reclaiming Artificial Wombs from Anti-abortion Discourse'. *Catalyst: Feminism, Theory, Technoscience* 6, no. 1 (2020): 1–15.

Huang, Zhelan, Tiantian Xiao and Wenhao Zhou. 'Artificial Womb: A Paradigm Shift for Saving Extremely Premature Infants'. *Chinese Medical Journal* 136, no. 14 (2023): 1759–61.

Hughes, Emma, and Jenny Kitzinger. 'Science Fiction Fears: An Analysis of How People Use Science Fiction in Discussing Risk and Emerging Science and Technology'. *Social Contexts and Responses to Risk Network (SCARR)*, Working Paper no. 28, 2008.

Hughes, Fiona, *Kant's Critique of Aesthetic Judgement*. London: Continuum, 2010.

Hughes, James J., and John D. Lantos. 'Medical Ethics Through the Star Trek Lens'. *Literature and Medicine* 20, no. 1 (2001): 26–38.

Hunter, Philip. 'Exogestation for Treating Premature Births and Congenital Diseases: Artificial Womb Technology Edges Toward First Trials in Humans'. *EMBO Reports* 25, no. 1 (2024): 17–20.

Hurley-Powell, Meghan. '"We're Never Trapped by Power": A Plurality of Feminist Resistance in Octavia Butler's Dawn'. *Journal of Literature, Culture and Literary Translation* 10, no. 1 (2019): 1–19.

Huxley, Aldous. *Brave New World*. London: Chatto and Windus, 1932.

Immega, Guy. *Super-Earth Mother: The AI that Engineered a Brave New World*. Calgary, Alberta: EDGE-Lite, 2023.

Inhorn, Marcia C. *Local Babies, Global Science: Gender, Religion and In Vitro Fertilization in Egypt*. New York: Routledge, 2003.

Jacobson, Daniel. 'Sir Philip Sydney's Dilemma: On the Ethical Treatment of Narrative Art'. *Journal of Aesthetics and Art Criticism* 54, no. 4 (1996): 327–36.

James, Henry. 'The Art of Fiction', in *Partial Portraits*, Henry James (ed.), 375–408. London: Macmillan and Co., Limited, 1899.

Jameson, Fredric. *Archaeologies of the Future: The Desire Called Utopia and Other Science Fiction*. London: Verso, 2005.

Jameson, Fredric. *Brecht and Method*. London: Verso, 1998.

Jameson, Fredric. 'Progress versus Utopia; Or, Can We Imagine the Future?' *Science Fiction Studies* 9, no. 2 (1982): 147–58.

Jasanoff, Sheila. 'Future Imperfect: Science, Technology, and the Imaginations of Modernity', in *Dreamscapes of Modernity: Sociotechnical Imaginaries and the Fabrication of Power*. Sheila Jasanoff and Kim Sang-Hyun (eds). Chicago: University of Chicago Press, 2015, 1–47.

Jay, Martin. 'In the Realm of the Senses: An Introduction'. *American Historical Review* 116, no. 2 (2011): 307–15.

Jesser, Nancy. 'Blood, Genes and Gender in Octavia Butler's *Kindred* and *Dawn*'. *Extrapolation* 43, no. 1 (2002): 36–61.

Johns, Alessa. 'Feminism and Utopia', in *The Cambridge Companion to Utopian Literature*. Gregory Claeys (ed.), 174–99. Cambridge: Cambridge University Press, 2010.

Johnson, Tess, and Elizabeth Chloe Romanis. 'The Relationship between Speculation and Translation in Bioethics: Methods and Methodologies'. *Monash Bioethics Review* 41 (Suppl 1) (2023): S1–S19.

Johnstone, Megan-Jane. 'Ethics and Ectogenesis'. *Australian Nursing Journal* 33, no. 11 (2010): 33.

Jones, Nancy C. 'Scientism or Luddism: Is Informed Ethical Possible?' *American Journal of Bioethics* 4, no. 1 (2004): 18–20.

Jordan, Monika. 'The Post-Dobbs World: How the Implementation of Fetal Personhood Laws Will Affect In Vitro Fertilization'. *UIC Law Review* 57, no. 2 (2024): 249–90.

Jurecic, Ann, and Daniel Marchalik. 'From Literature to Medicine: Dr Frankenstein's Bioethical Experiment'. *Lancet* 386 (2015): 1223.

Kabata, Faith, and Donrich Thaldar. 'The Human Genome as the Common Heritage of Mankind'. *Frontiers in Genetics* 14 (2023): 1282515.

Kaczor, Christopher. 'Artificial Wombs and Embryo Adoption', in *The Ethics of Embryo Adoption and the Catholic Tradition: Moral Arguments, Economic Reality and Social Analysis*. Sarah-Vaughan Brakman and Darlene Fozard Weaver (eds), 307–22. Dordrecht: Springer, 2007.

Kant, Immanuel. 'Groundwork of the Metaphysics of Morals', in *Practical Philosophy.* Mary Gregor (trans), 37–108. Cambridge: Cambridge University Press, 1996.

Kass, Leon. 'Forbidding Science: Some Beginning Reflections'. *Science and Engineering Ethics* 15 (2009): 271–282.

Kass, Leon. 'The Wisdom of Repugnance'. *The New Republic* 216, no. 22 (1997): 17–26.

Kavanagh, Terry (writer), Roger Cruz (penciller), Rud LaRosa and Wellington Diaz (inkers). 'Breeding Ground', *X-man,* Volume 1, #-1. New York: Marvel Comics Group, 1997.

Kendal, Evie. 'Desire, Duty, and Discrimination: Is There an Ethical Way to Select Human's for Noah's Ark?' in *Reclaiming Space: Progressive and Multicultural Visions of Space Exploration*, J. S. J. Schwartz, Linda Billings and Erika Nesvold (eds), 289–302. Oxford: Oxford University Press, 2023.

Kendal, Evie. 'Form, Function, Perception, and Reception: Visual Bioethics and the Artificial Womb'. *Yale Journal of Biology and Medicine* 95 (2022): 371–7.

Kendal, Evie. 'Ectogenesis and the Ethics of New Reproductive Technologies for Space Exploration' in *Transhumanism: Entering an Era of Bodyhacking and Radical Human Modification*. Emma Tumilty and Michele Battle-Fisher (eds), 211–26. Cham: Springer, 2022.

Kendal, Evie. 'Ectogenesis for Space Exploration'. in *eLS* 2 (2021): 1–5.

Kendal, Evie. 'The Use of Free Indirect Discourse in J.R. Ward's *Black Dagger Brotherhood* series'. *Colloquy: Text, Theory, Critique* 38 (2019): 20–43.

Kendal, Evie. *Equal Opportunity and the Case for State Sponsored Ectogenesis*. Basingstoke: Palgrave Macmillan, 2015.

Kendal, Evie. 'Utopian Visions of "Making People": Science Fiction and Debates on Cloning, Ectogenesis, Genetic Engineering, and Genetic Discrimination', in *Biopolitics and Utopia: An Interdisciplinary Reader*. Patricia Stapleton and Andrew Byers (eds), 89–117. New York: Palgrave Macmillan, 2015.

Kendal, Evie, and Julian J. Koplin. 'The Moral Superiority of Bioengineered Wombs and Ectogenesis for Absolute Uterine Factor Infertility'. *Cambridge Quarterly of Healthcare Ethics* 31, no. 1 (2022): 73–82.

Kennedy, Susan, and Lawrence Nelson. 'A Different Take on the Law and Ethics of AWT'. *American Journal of Bioethics* 23, no. 5 (2023): 92–4.

Khulbe, Yashita, Shiva Gupta, Binish Javed, Ahmad Neyazi and Bijaya K. Padhi. 'Artificial Womb: Opportunities and Challenges for Public Health'. *International Journal of Surgery* 109, no. 3 (2023): 618–19.

Kimberly, Laura L., and Gwendolyn P. Quinn. 'Toward a Broader Conception of Equity in Artificial Womb Technology'. *American Journal of Bioethics* 23, no. 5 (2023): 114–16.

Kin, Curtis A. 'Coming Soon to the "Genetic Supermarket" Near You'. *Stanford Law Review* 48, no. 6 (1996): 1573–604.

Kincaid, Paul. 'On the Origins of Genre'. *Extrapolation* 44, no. 4 (2003): 409–19.

Kingma, Elselijn, and Suki Finn. 'Neonatal Incubator or Artificial Womb? Distinguishing Ectogestation and Ectogenesis Using the Metaphysics of Pregnancy'. *Bioethics* 34, no. 4 (2020): 354–63.

Kirby, David A. 'The Devil in Our DNA: A Brief History of Eugenics in Science Fiction Films', *Literature and Medicine* 26, no. 1 (2007): 83–108.

Kirby, David A.'The New Eugenics in Cinema: Genetic Determinism and Gene Therapy in "GATTACA"'. *Science Fiction Studies* 27, no. 2 (2000): 193–215.

Kitzinger, Jenny. 'Questioning the Sci-Fi Alibi: A Critique of How "Science Fiction Fears" Are Used to Explain Away Public Concerns about Risk'. *Journal of Risk Research* 13, no. 1 (2010): 73–86.

Klass, Perri. 'The Artificial Womb Is Born'. *The New York Times* online, 29 September 1996. Accessed 12 November 2014. http://www.nytimes.com/1996/09/29/magazine/the-artificial-womb-is-born.html?

Köppe, Tilmann, and Tom Kindt. 'Unreliable Narration with a Narrator and without'. *Journal of Literary Theory* 5, no. 1 (2011): 81–94.

Kozlov, Max. 'Human Trials of Artificial Wombs Could Start Soon. Here's What You Need to Know'. *Nature*, 14 September 2023. Accessed 22 January 2024. https://www.nature.com/articles/d41586-023-02901-1

Krendel, Alexandra, and Mike Ryder. 'Role of Science Fiction in Conceptualising the Reproductive Future: A Linguistic and Literary Perspective'. *Medical Humanities* (2025). DOI: 10.1136/medhum-2024-013207

Kristeva, Julia. *Powers of Horror: An Essay on Abjection*. Leon S. Roudiez (trans). New York: Columbia University Press, 1982.

Kukora, Stephanie K., George B. Mychaliska and Elliott Mark Weiss. 'Ethical Challenges for First-in-Human Trials of the Artificial Placenta and Artificial Womb: Not All Technologies are Created Equally, Ethically'. *Journal of Perinatology* 43 (2023): 1337–42.

Kundu, Pritha. '"The Doctor's Dilemma" and Bioethics in Literature: An Interdisciplinary Approach'. *Janus Head* 16, no. 1 (2018): 119–37.

Kyle XY. Created by Eric Bress and J. Mackye Gruber. Burbank, California: ABC Studios: 2006–2009.

Lahl, Jennifer C. 'Caveat Emptor'. *American Journal of Bioethics* 4, no. 1 (2004): 20–1.

Lake, Christina Bieber. *Prophets of the Posthuman: American Fiction, Biotechnology, and the Ethics of Personhood*. Indiana: University of Notre Dame Press, 2013.

Lallanilla, Mark. 'Human Embryos Created without Egg or Sperm in Controversial Breakthrough'. *New York Post*, 15 June 2023. Accessed 15 February 2024. https://nypost.com/2023/06/15/human-embryos-created-without-egg-or-sperm-in-controversial-breakthrough/

Langford, Sarah. 'An End to Abortion? A Feminist Critique of the "Ectogenetic Solution" to Abortion'. *Women's Studies International Forum* 31 (2008): 263–9.

Lanser, Susan S. 'Toward a Feminist Narratology'. *Style* 20, no. 3 (1986): 341–63.

Lanser, Susan S. *The Narrative Act: Point of View in Prose Fiction*. New Jersey: Princeton University Press, 1981.

Lanser, Susan S. 'Toward (a Queerer and) More (Feminist) Narratology', in *Narrative Theory Unbound: Queer and Feminist Interventions*. Robyn Warhol and Susan S. Lanser (eds), 23–42. Columbus: Ohio State University Press, 2015.

Lantos, John D., and Annie Janvier. 'The Dilemmas of Artificial Wombs: Conventional Ethics and Science Fiction'. *American Journal of Bioethics* 23, no. 5 (2023): 82–5.

Latimer, Heather. 'Reproductive Technologies, Fetal Icons, and Genetic Freaks: Shelley Jackson's *Patchwork Girl* and the Limits and Possibilities of Donna Haraway's Cyborg'. *Modern Fiction Studies* 57, no. 2 (2011): 318–35.

Lauritzen, Paul. 'Visual Bioethics'. *American Journal of Bioethics* 8, no. 12 (2008): 50–6.

Le Guin, Ursula K. *The Left Hand of Darkness*. New York: Ace Books, 1969.

Lesnik-Oberstein, Karin. *Children's Literature: Criticism and the Fictional Child*. Oxford: Clarendon Press, 1994.

Levitas, Ruth. *Utopia as Method: The Imaginary Reconstruction of Society*. Basingstoke: Palgrave Macmillan, 2013.

Lewis, Sophie. *Full Surrogacy Now: Feminism Against Family*. London: Verso Books, 2019.

Lindemann, Hilde. 'In the Matter of Stories'. *Perspectives in Biology and Medicine* 60, no. 1 (2017): 93–102.

Lindloff, Thomas R., Kelly Coyle, and Debra Grodin. 'Is There a Text in This Audience? Science Fiction and Interpretive Schism', in *Theorizing Fandom: Fans, Subculture and Identity*. Cheryl Harris and Alison Alexander (eds), 219–47. New Jersey: Hampton Press, 1998.

Livingston, Dennis. 'The Biology of Utopia: Science Fiction Perspectives on Ectogenesis', in *The Custom-made Child? Women-centred Perspectives*. Helen B. Holmes, Betty B. Hoskins and Michael Gross (eds), 281–9. New Jersey: Humana Press, 1981.

Lo, Kinling. 'China's Gene-editing 'Frankenstein' Jailed for Three Years in Modified Baby Case'. *South China Morning Post*, 30 December 2019. Accessed 19 February 2024. https://www.scmp.com/news/china/science/article/3043894/chinas-gene-editing-frankenstein-jailed-3-years-modified-baby

Lobdell, Scott (writer), R. B. Silva (illustrator) and Rob Lean (illustrator). 'Incubation'. DC New 52 *Superboy*, volume 1 #1–7. Burbank, California: DC Comics, 2011.

Lomotey-Nakon, Leah, and Elizabeth Lanphier. 'Expanding the Frame: An Afrofuturist Response to Artificial Womb Technology'. *American Journal of Bioethics* 23, no. 5 (2023): 99–101.

Lowentrout, Peter. 'The "Metamorphoses" of Darko Suvin: Final Synthesis or Dogged Antithesis?' *Foundation*, no. 42 (1988): 37–45.

Maher, JaneMaree. 'A Pregnant Man in the Movies: The Visual Politics of Reproduction'. *Continuum: Journal of Media & Cultural Studies* 22, no. 2 (2008): 279–88.

Maher, JaneMaree. 'Visibly Pregnant: Toward a Placental Body'. *Feminist Review* 72 (2002): 95–107.

Mann, Justin Louis. 'Pessimistic Futurism: Survival and Reproduction in Octavia Butler's *Dawn*'. *Feminist Theory* 19, no. 1 (2017): 61–76.

Mascarenhas, Lauren, and Melissa Alonso. 'Alabama State Senator Proposes Bill to Protect IVF Medical Providers'. *CNN*, 27 February 2024. Accessed 28 February 2024. https://edition.cnn.com/2024/02/27/us/ivf-ruling-impact-other-states/index.html

Mason, Chris. 'Making People: Today's Wariness of Reproductive Technologies Stems from Myths, Legends and Hollywood'. *Nature* 471, no. 7338 (2011): 297–9.

Maienschein, Jane. 'Part II: What's in a Name: Embryos, Clones, and Stem Cells'. *American Journal of Bioethics* 2, no. 1 (2002): 12–19.

McLeod, Ken. 'GATTACA', in *The Influence of Imagination: Essays on Science Fiction and Fantasy as Agents of Social Change*. Lee Easton and Randy Schroeder (eds.), 174–6. Jefferson: McFarland & Company, 2007.

Menadue, Christopher Benjamin, Kristi Giselsson and David Guez. 'An Empirical Revision of the Definition of Science Fiction: It Is All in the Techne…'. *SAGE Open* 10, no. 4 (2020): 1–18.

Mendeloff, John. 'Politics and Bioethical Commissions: "Muddling Through" and the "Slippery Slope"'. *Journal of Health Politics, Policy and Law* 10, no. 1 (1985): 81–92.

Mercurio, Mark R., and Kelly M. Werner. 'Thinking Inside the Bag: Patient Selection, Framing the Ethical Discourse, and the Importance of Terminology in Artificial Womb Technology'. *American Journal of Bioethics* 23, no. 5 (2023): 79–82.

Meyers, Diana. 'The Rush to Motherhood: Pronatalist Discourse and Women's Autonomy'. *Signs* 26, no. 3 (2001): 735–73.

Miéville, China. 'Cognition as Ideology: A Dialectic of SF Theory', in *Red Planets: Marxism and Science Fiction*. Mark Bould and China Miéville (eds). London: Pluto, 2009, 231–48.

Mills, Catherine. 'Images and Emotion in Abortion Debates'. *American Journal of Bioethics* 8, no. 12 (2008): 61–2.

Millum, Joseph. 'The Foundation of the Child's Right to an Open Future'. *Journal of Social Philosophy* 45, no. 4 (2014): 522–38.

Milner, Andrew. 'Resources for a Journey of Hope: Raymond Williams on Utopia and Science Fiction'. *Cultural Sociology* 10, no. 4 (2016): 415–30.

Milner, Andrew. 'Colonialism and the Emergence of Science Fiction by John Rieder (review)'. *Science Fiction Film and Television* 6, no. 1 (2013): 138–42.

Milner, Andrew. *Literature, Culture and Society*, 2nd edition. London: Routledge, 2004.

Milner, Andrew, J. R. Burgmann, Rjurik Davidson and Susan Cousin. 'Ice, Fire, Flood: Science Fiction and the Anthropocene'. *Thesis Eleven* 131, no. 1 (2015): 12–27.

Morgan, Lynn M., and Meredith W. Michaels. 'Part II: Manipulating the Fetal Image', in *Fetal Subjects, Feminist Positions*, Lynn M. Morgan and Meredith W. Michaels (eds), 99–100. Philadelphia: University of Pennsylvania Press, 1999.

Morgan, S. Philip, Suzanne Shanahan and Whitney Welsh. 'Brave New Worlds: Philosophy, Politics, and Science in Human Biotechnology'. *Population and Development Review*, vol. 31, no. 1 (2005): 127–41.

Morrison, Grant (writer), Andy Kubert (penciller) and Jesse Delperdang (inker). 'Batman in Bethlehem', *Batman*, Volume 1 #666, in *Batman and Son*. Burbank, California: DC Comics, 2007.

Moylan, Tom. *Scraps of the Untainted Sky: Science Fiction, Utopia, Dystopia*. Boulder: Westview Press, 2000.

Moylan, Tom. *Demand the Impossible: Science Fiction and the Utopian Imagination*. London: Methuen, 1986.

Mullin, Amy. 'Moral Defects, Aesthetic Defects, and the Imagination'. *Journal of Aesthetics and Art Criticism* 62, no. 3 (2004): 249–61.

Murcott, Anne. 'Public Beliefs about GM Foods: More on the Makings of a Considered Sociology'. *Medical Anthropology Quarterly* 15, no. 1 (2001): 9–19.

Murphy, Julien S. 'Is Pregnancy Necessary? Feminist Concerns about Ectogenesis'. *Hypatia* 4, no. 3 (1989): 66–84.

Nabuurs, Joyce, Anouk Heltzel, Willemine Willems and Frank Kupper. 'Crafting the Future of the Artificial Womb – Speculative Design as a Tool for Public Engagement with Emerging Technologies'. *Futures* 151 (2023): 103184

National Health and Medical Research Council. 'NHMRC Opens Public Consultation on Draft Ethical Guidelines for Xenotransplantation Research'. NHMRC website. Accessed 9 July 2016. https://www.nhmrc.gov.au/media/releases/2016/nhmrc-opens-public-consultation-draft-ethical-guidelines-xenotransplantation

Nelson, Hilde Lindemann. 'Introduction: How to Do Things with Stories', in *Stories and Their Limits: Narrative Approaches to Bioethics*. Hilde L. Nelson (ed.). London: Routledge, 1997, vii–xx.

Nickel, Philip J. 'Horror and the Idea of Everyday Life: On Skeptical Threats in *Psycho* and *The Birds*', in *The Philosophy of Horror*. Thomas Fahey (ed.) Kentucky: The University Press of Kentucky, 2010, 14–32.

Nierenberg, Danielle. 'The Health Hazards of Being Female', in *Correcting Gender Myopia: Gender Equity, Women's Welfare, and the Environment*. Washington: World Watch Institute, 2002, 29–37.

Niven, Larry, Jerry Pournelle and Steven Barnes. *The Dragons of Heorot*. London: Gollancz, 1995.

Nordmann, Alfred. *Wittgenstein's Tractatus: An Introduction*. Cambridge: Cambridge University Press, 2005.

Nussbaum, Martha C. ' "Finely Aware and Richly Responsible": Literature and the Moral Imagination', in *Love's Knowledge: Essays on Philosophy and Literature*. New York: Oxford University Press, 1990, 148–67.

Nüsslein-Volhard, Christiane. 'Manipulating the Human Embryo'. *USA Today* (2011): 30.

O'Brien, Mary. *The Politics of Reproduction*. London: Routledge & Kegan Paul, 1981.

O'Donovan, Laura, Nicola Jane Williams and Stephen Wilkinson. 'Ethical and Policy Issues Raised by Uterus Transplants'. *British Medical Bulletin* 131, no. 1 (2019): 19–28.

Okoye, Florence. 'Afrofuturism as Intersectional Transhumanism'. Presentation at *Techno Resistance and Black Future Festival*, Goldsmiths, London, 2017. Accessed 18 March 2024. https://finokoye.files.wordpress.com/2019/08/af_as_it_presentation.pdf

Olausson, Michael, Liza Johannesson, Daniel Brattgård, Cesar Diaz-Garcia, Cecilia Lundmark, Klaus Groth, Janusz Marcickiewizc, Anders Enskog, Randa Akouri, Andreas Tzakis, Xavier Rogiers, Per Olof Janson and Mats Brännström. 'Ethics of Uterus Transplantation with Live Donors'. *Fertility and Sterility* 102, no. 1 (2014): 40–3.

Oltean, Stefan. 'A Survey of the Pragmatic and Referential Functions of Free Indirect Discourse'. *Poetics Today* 14, no. 4 (1993): 691–714.

Osherow, Michele. 'The Dawn of a New Lilith: Revisionary Mythmaking in Women's Science Fiction'. *NWSA Journal* 12, no. 1 (2000): 68–83.

Otway, Nick, and Megan Ellis. 'Construction and Test of an Artificial Uterus for Ex Situ Development of Shark Embryos'. *Zoo Biology* 31 (2012): 197–205.

Overall, Christine. *Ethics and Human Reproduction: A Feminist Analysis*. London: Routledge, 1987.

Oxley, Julinna C. 'Liberal Feminism', in *Just the Arguments: 100 of the Most Important Arguments in Western Philosophy*. Michael Bruce and Steven Barbone (eds), 258–62. Chichester: Blackwell Publishing, 2011.

Partridge, Emily A., Marcus G. Davey, Matthew A. Hornick, Patrick E. McGovern, Ali Y. Mejaddam, Jesse D. Vrecenak, Carmen Mesas-Burgos, Aliza Olive, Robert C. Caskey, Theodore R. Weiland, Jiancheng Han, Alexander J. Schupper, James T. Connelly, Kevin C. Dysart, Jack Rychik, Holly L. Hedrick, William H. Peranteau and Alan W. Flake. 'An Extra-uterine System to Physiologically Support the Extreme Premature Lamb'. *Nature Communications* 8 (2017). DOI: 10.1038/ncomms15112.

Paul, Lissa. 'Sex and the Children's Book', *The Lion and the Unicorn* 29, no. 2 (2005): 222–35.

Pence, Gregory. 'What's So Good about Natural Motherhood? (In Praise of Unnatural Gestation)', in *Ectogenesis: Artificial Womb Technology and the Future of Human Reproduction*. Scott Gelfand and John Shook (eds), 77–88. New York: Rodopi, 2006.

Pence, Gregory. *Who's Afraid of Human Cloning?* Lanham: Rowman and Littlefield Publishers, 1998.

Petchesky, Rosalind Pollack. 'Fetal Images: The Power of Visual Culture in the Politics of Reproduction'. *Feminist Studies* 13, no. 2 (1987): 263–92.

Peters, Ted, and Gaymon Bennett, Jr. 'Stem Cell Research and the Claim of the Other in the Human Subject'. *Dialog: A Journal of Theology* 43, no. 3 (2004): 184–204.

Peterson, Susan Rae. 'The Politics of Prenatal Diagnosis: A Feminist Ethical Analysis', in *The Custom-Made Child? Women-Centred Perspectives*. Helen B. Holmes, Betty B. Hoskins and Michael Gross (eds), 95–104. New Jersey: Humana Press, 1981.

Piercy, Marge. *Woman on the Edge of Time*. New York: Ballantine Books, 1976.

Platt, John. 'Artificial Uterus Could Save Grey Nurse Shark from Extinction'. *Scientific American*, 18 February 2009. Accessed 22 January 2024. https://blogs.scientificamerican.com/extinction-countdown/artificial-uterus-could-save-grey-nurse-shark-from-extinction/

Prince, Gerald. 'Narrative Analysis and Narratology'. *New Literary History* 13, no. 2 (1982): 179–88.

Rabkin, Eric S. 'Science Fiction and Bioethical Knowledge', in *Bioethics and Biolaw through Literature*. Daniela Carpi (ed.), 137–48. Berlin: De Gruyter, 2011.

Radford, Colin, and Michael Weston. 'How Can We Be Moved by the Fate of Anna Karenina?' *Proceedings of the Aristotelian Society, Supplementary Volumes* 49 (1975): 67–93.

Racine, Eric, Tristana Martin Rubio, Jennifer Chandler, Cynthia Forlini and Jayne Lucke. 'The Value and Pitfalls of Speculation about Science and Technology in Bioethics: The Case of Cognitive Enhancement'. *Medicine, Health Care and Philosophy* 17, no. 3 (2014): 325–38.

Räsänen, Joona. 'Ectogenesis, Abortion and a Right to the Death of the Fetus'. *Bioethics* 31, no. 9 (2017): 697–702.

Raymond, Janice G. 'Reproductive Gifts and Gift Giving: The Altruistic Woman', in *Life Choices: A Hastings Center Introduction to Bioethics,* 2nd edition. Joseph H. Howell and William Frederick Sale (eds), 395–406. Washington D.C.: Georgetown University Press, 2000.

Raymond, Janice G. 'Maternal Environments and Ejaculatory Fathers: New Definitions of Motherhood and Fatherhood', in *Women as Wombs: Reproductive Technologies and the Battle over Women's Freedom*. 29–75. Melbourne: Spinifex Press Pty., 1994.

Rayne, Elizabeth. 'Brave New World Is Being Reinvented with Synthetic Embryos–and the Right Reasons'. *Syfy*, 1 May 2021. Accessed 15 February 2024. https://www.syfy.com/syfy-wire/brave-new-world-reinvented-with-synthetic-embryos

Renault, Gregory. 'Science Fiction as Cognitive Estrangement: Darko Suvin and the Marxist Critique of Mass Culture'. *Discourse* 2 (1980): 113–41.

Rieder, John. 'Review: Utopia, SF, and the Ideology of Form'. *Science Fiction Studies* 42, no. 3 (2015): 566–73.

Rieder, John. 'On Defining SF, or Not: Genre Theory, SF, and History'. *Science Fiction Studies* 37, no. 2 (2010): 191–209.

Rifkin, Jeremy. 'Evolution's Pregnant Pause: Artificial Wombs'. *Los Angeles Times*, 21 January 2002, Accessed 24 January 2024, https://www.latimes.com/archives/la-xpm-2002-jan-21-oe-rifkin21-story.html

Rifkin, Jeremy. *The Biotech Century: Harnessing the Gene and Remaking the World*. New York: Putnam, 1998.

Robertson, Benjamin J. 'Freedman, Carl. Art and Idea in the Novels of China Miéville. Canterbury, UK: Gylphi, 2015. 183 pp. Paperback. ISBN 978-1-78024-030-5. $29.99; Edwards, Caroline and Tony Venezia, eds. China Miéville: Critical Essays. Canterbury, UK: Gylphi, 2015. 296 pp. Paperback. ISBN 978-1-78024-027-5. $29.99 [review]'. *Journal of the Fantastic in the Arts* 27, no. 2 (2016): 364–84.

Robins, Rosemary. 'Public and Popular Representations of "Frankenscience"'. *Social Studies of Science* 29, no. 2 (1999): 295–301.

Roesner, Nina. 'Beyond a Medicalized View of Reproduction: Recentering Pregnant People in the Ethics of Ectogenesis'. *American Journal of Bioethics* 23, no. 5 (2023): 102–4.

Romanis, Elizabeth Chloe. 'Equality-Enhancing Potential of Novel Forms of Assisted Gestation: Perspectives of Reproductive Rights Advocates'. *Bioethics* 37 (2023): 637–46.

Romanis, Elizabeth Chloe. 'The Ethical and Legal Status of "Fetonates" or "Gestatelings"'. *American Journal of Bioethics* 23, no. 5 (2023): 90–92.

Romanis, Elizabeth Chloe. 'Artificial Womb Technology and Clinical Translation: Innovative Treatment or Medical Research?' Bioethics 34, no. 4 (2020): 392–402.

Romanis, Elizabeth Chloe. 'Challenging the "Born Alive" Threshold: Fetal Surgery, Artificial Wombs, and the English Approach to Legal Personhood'. *Medical Law Review* 28, no. 1 (2020): 93–123.

Romanis, Elizabeth Chloe. 'Artificial Womb Technology and the Significance of Birth: Why Gestatelings Are Not Newborns (or Fetuses)'. *Journal of Medical Ethics* 45, no. 11 (2019): 728–31.

Romanis, Elizabeth Chloe, and Victoria Adkins. 'Artificial Placentas, Pregnancy Loss and Loss-Sensitive Care'. *Journal of Medical Ethics* 50, no. 5 (2024): 299–307.

Romanis, Elizabeth Chloe, Seppe Segers and Ben D. de Jong. 'Value Sensitive Design and the Artificial Placenta'. *Journal of Medical Ethics* (2024). DOI: 10.1136/jme-2024-110066.

Rothman, Barbara Katz. *A Bun in the Oven: How the Food and Birth Movements Resist Industrialization*. New York: NYU Press, 2016.

Rowland, Robyn. 'Technology and Motherhood: Reproductive Choice Reconsidered'. *Signs* 12, no. 3 (1987): 512–28.

Rudy, Kathy. 'Ethics, Reproduction, Utopia: Gender and Childbearing in "Woman on the Edge of Time" and "The Left Hand of Darkness"'. *NWSA Journal* 9, no. 1 (1997): 22–38.

Russ, Joanna. 'Towards an Aesthetic of Science Fiction'. *Science Fiction Studies* 2 (1976): 112–19.

Russell, Brenda, Debra Oswald and MaryKate Cotter. 'What Makes a Liberal Feminist? Identifying Predictors of Heterosexual Women and Men's Liberal Feminist Ideology'. *Analyses of Social Issues and Public Policy* 24, no. 1 (2024): 241–60.

Sanz Alonso, Irene. 'Science Fiction Magnifying Mirrors: Octavia Butler's *Dawn* and the Ethics of Genetic Manipulation'. *Proceedings of the 31st AEDEAN Conference* (2008): 881–8.

Sargent, Lyman Tower. 'Authority and Utopia: Utopianism in Political Thought'. *Polity Journal* 14, no. 4 (1982): 565–84.

Sasaki, Kaori. 'Bioethics Between Imaginary and Reality: Tracing Science Fiction and Its Shaping of Transplant Medicine Protocols in Japan'. *East Asian Science, Technology and Society: An International Journal* 13, no. 1 (2019): 77–99.

Savulescu, Julian. 'Procreative Beneficence: Why We Should Select the Best Children'. *Bioethics* 15, no. 5–6 (2001): 413–26.

Schiller, Fred (writer), Tony Akins (penciller) and Jim Brozman (inker). 'Factories'. *The Terminator* #11. Chicago: Now Comics, 1989.

Schiller, Fred (writer), Tony Akins (penciller) and Jim Brozman (inker). 'Night Convoy'. *The Terminator* #12. Chicago: Now Comics, 1989.

Schlickers, Sabine. 'Focalization, Ocularization and Auricularization in Film and Literature', in *Point of View, Perspective, and Focalization: Modeling Mediation in Narrative*. Peter Hühn, Wolf Schmid and Jörg Schönert (eds). Berlin: Walter de Gruyter (2009): 243–58.

Schmid, Wolf. *Narratology: An Introduction*, Alexander Starritt (trans). Berlin: Walter de Gruyer, 2010.

Schuck, A. R. T., and C. H. de Vreese. 'Between Risk and Opportunity: News Framing and its Effects on Public Support for EU Enlargement'. *European Journal of Communication* 21, no. 1 (2006): 5–32.

Schuelke, Gertrude. 'Slipping' in Indirect Discourse'. *American Speech* 33, no. 2 (1958): 90–8.

Schultz, Jessica H. 'Development of Ectogenesis: How Will Artificial Wombs Affect the Legal Status of a Fetus or Embryo?' *Chicago-Kent Law Review* 84 (2010): 877–906.

Sedgwick, Helen. *The Growing Season*. London: Harvill Seeker, 2017.

Segers, Seppe. 'The Path Toward Ectogenesis: Looking Beyond the Technical Challenges'. *BMC Medical Ethics* 22 (2021): 59.

Segers, Seppe, and Dorian Accoe. 'The Ethics of Ectogestative Technology – Telling Science from Science Fiction'. *JAMA Pediatrics* 177, no. 10 (2023): 1110.

Segers, Seppe, and Elizabeth Chloe Romanis. 'Ethical, Translational, and Legal Issues Surrounding the Novel Adoption of Ectogestative Technologies'. *Risk Management and Healthcare Policy* 15 (2022): 2207–20.

Segers, Seppe, Guido Pennings and Heidi Mertens. 'The Ethics of Ectogenesis-aided Foetal Treatment'. *Bioethics* 34 (2020): 364–70.

Seiple, Samantha, and Todd Seiple. *Mutants, Clones and Killer Corn: Unlocking the Secrets of Biotechnology*. Minneapolis: Lerner Publications Company, 2005.

Shah, Aakash M. 'FDA on the Verge of Approving Human Clinical Trial for Artificial Womb'. *Artificial Organs* 47 (2023): 1683–4.

Shapshay, Sandra. 'Lifting the Genetic Veil of Ignorance: Is There Anything Really Unjust about Gattacan Society?' in *Bioethics at the Movies*. Sandra Shapshay (ed.). Baltimore: The John Hopkins University Press, 2009, 87–101.

Sharvit, Yael. 'The Puzzle of Free Indirect Discourse'. *Linguistics and Philosophy* 31 (2008): 353–95.

Shelley, Mary. *Frankenstein: Or, the Modern Prometheus*. London: Lackington, Hughes, Harding, Mavor & Jones, 1818.

Shen, Dan. 'Stylistics, Narratology, and Point of View: Partiality, Complementarity, and A New Definition'. *Style* 57, no. 4 (2023): 415–39.

Sibley, Mulford Q. 'Apology for Utopia II: Utopia and Politics'. *Journal of Politics* 2, No 2 (1940): 165–88.

Silver, Lee M. *Remaking Eden: Cloning, Genetic Engineering and the Future of Humankind?* London: Phoenix Giant, 1998.

Silver, Lee M. 'Genetics Goes to Hollywood'. *Nature Genetics* 17 (1997): 260.

Silverman, William A. 'Incubator-Baby Side Shows'. *Pediatrics* 64, no. 2 (1979): 127–41.

Simonstein, Frida, and Michal Mashiach-Eizenberg. 'The Artificial Womb: A Pilot Study Considering People's Views on the Artificial Womb and Ectogenesis in Israel'. *Cambridge Quarterly of Healthcare Ethics* 18 (2009): 87–94.

Singer, Peter, and Deane Wells. 'Ectogenesis', in *Ectogenesis: Artificial Womb Technology and the Future of Human Reproduction*. Scott Gelfand and John Shook (eds), 9–26. New York: Rodopi, 2006.

Slonczewski, Joan. 'An Interview with Joan Slonczewski', in *Posthuman Biopolitics: The Science Fiction of Joan Slonczewski*. Bruce Clarke (ed.), 1–16. Cham: Palgrave Macmillan, 2020.

Smajdor, Anna. 'In Defense of Ectogenesis'. *Cambridge Quarterly of Healthcare Ethics* 21, no. 1 (2012): 90–103.

Smajdor, Anna. 'The Moral Imperative for Ectogenesis'. *Cambridge Quarterly Healthcare Ethics* 16, no. 3 (2007): 336–45.

Smith, George P. II. 'Intimations of Immortality: Clones, Cyrons and the Law'. *U.N.S.W. Law Journal* 6 (1983): 119–32.

Smith, Wesley J. 'About Those "Synthetic Embryos"'. *National Review*, 8 August 2022. Accessed 15 February 2024. https://www.nationalreview.com/corner/about-those-synthetic-embryos/

Smookler, Jennifer. 'Feminism, Liberal Democracy and the Politics of Inclusion and Exclusion'. *Political Studies Association – UK Annual Conference Proceedings*, University of London (2000): 1–13.

So, Derek. 'From Goodness to Good Looks: Changing Images of Human Germline Genetic Modification'. *Bioethics* 36 (2022): 556–68.

Spencer, Kathleen L. '"The Red Sun is High, the Blue Low": Towards a Stylistic Description of Science Fiction ("Le soleil rouge est au zénith, le soleil bleu se couche": vers une description stylistique de la SF)'. *Science Fiction Studies* 10, no. 1 (1983): 35–49.

Splice. [Film] Directed by Vincenzo Natali. Neuilly-sur-Seine, France: Gaumont, 2009.

Squier, Susan M. *Liminal Lives: Imagining the Human at the Frontiers of Biomedicine*. Durham: Duke University Press (2004).

Squier, Susan M. 'Negotiating Boundaries: From Assisted Reproduction to Assisted Replication', in *Playing Dolly: Technocultural Formations, Fantasies, & Fictions of Assisted Reproduction*. E. Ann Kaplan and Susan Squier (eds), 101–15. New Brunswick: Rutgers University Press, 1999.

Squier, Susan M. 'Reproducing the Posthuman Body: Ectogenetic Fetus, Surrogate Mother, Pregnant Man', in *Posthuman Bodies*. Judith Halberstam and Ira Livingston (eds), 113–32. Bloomington: Indiana University Press, 1995.

Squier, Susan M. *Babies in Bottles: Twentieth-Century Visions of Reproductive Technology*. New Brunswick: Rutgers University Press, 1994.

Stanton, Kate. 'Sounds Like Science Fiction'. *Pursuit*, 27 December 2017. Accessed 19 February 2024. https://pursuit.unimelb.edu.au/articles/sounds-like-science-fiction

Steiger, Eric. 'Not of Woman Born: How Ectogenesis Will Change the Way We View Viability, Birth, and the Status of the Unborn'. *Journal of Law and Health* 23, no. 2 (2010): 143–71.

Stellman, Jeanne, and Mary Sue Henifin. 'No Fertile Women Need Apply: Employment Discrimination and Reproductive Hazards in the Workplace', in *Biological Woman – The Convenient Myth: A Collection of Feminist Essays and a Comprehensive Bibliography*. Ruth Hubbard, Mary Sue Henifin and Barbara Fried (eds), 117–20. Cambridge: Schenkman Publishing, 1982.

Stephenson, Niamh, Catherine Mills and Kim McLeod. "Simply Providing Information': Negotiating the Ethical Dilemmas of Obstetric Ultrasound, Prenatal Testing and Selective Termination of Pregnancy'. *Feminism and Psychology* 27, no. 1 (2016): 72–91.

Stoesz, David. *A Poverty of Imagination: Bootstrap Capitalism, Sequel to Welfare Reform*. Wisconsin: Wisconsin University Press, 2000.

Stys, John C. 'Documentary Bioethics: Visual Narratives for Generations X and Y'. *Journal of Medical Humanities* 27, no. 1 (2006): 57–66.

Suvin, Darko. 'Centennial Politics: On Jameson on Brecht on Method'. *New Left Review*, no. 234 (1999): 127–140.

Suvin, Darko. Narrative Logic, Ideological Domination, and the Range of Science Fiction: A Hypothesis with a Historical Test (Logique narrative, dominate idéologique et l'éventail de la S-F: hypothèse et épreuve historique'. *Science Fiction Studies* 9, no. 1 (1982): 1–25.

Suvin, Darko. *Metamorphoses of Science Fiction: On the Poetics and History of a Literary Genre*. New Haven: Yale University Press, 1979.

Suvin, Darko. 'The State of the Art in Science Fiction Theory: Determining and Delimiting the Genre (Etat présent de la théorie de science-fiction: détermination et délimitation du genre)'. *Science Fiction Studies* 6, no. 1 (1979): 32–45.

Suvin, Darko. 'On What Is and Is Not an SF Narration: With a List of 101 Victorian Books That Should Be Excluded from SF Bibliographies'. *Science Fiction Studies* 5, no. 1 (1978): 45–57.

Suvin, Darko. 'Defining the Literary Genre of Utopia: Some Historical Semantics, Some Genology, a Proposal and a Plea'. *Studies in the Literary Imagination* 6 (1973): 121–45.

Szocik, Konrad. 'Humanity Should Colonise in Order to Survive But Not with Embryo Space Colonization'. *International Journal of Astrobiology* 20, no. 4 (2021): 319–22.

Takashima, Kyoko, Tomohide Ibuki and Keiichiro Yamamoto. 'Is the Mother's Decision to Opt for Artificial Womb Technology Always "Supererogatory"?' *American Journal of Bioethics* 23, no. 5 (2023): 119–21.

Terry, James S., and Peter C. Williams. 'Literature and Bioethics: The Tension in Goals and Styles'. *Literature and Medicine* 7 (1988): 1–21.

Testa, Giuliano, Greg J. McKenna, Anji Wall, Johanna Bayer, Anthony R. Gregg, Ann Marie Warren, Seung Hee S. Lee, Eric Martinez, Amar Gupta, Robert Gunby and Liza Johannesson. 'Uterus Transplant in Women with Absolute Uterine-Factor Infertility'. *JAMA* 332, no. 10 (2024): 817–24.

Thacker, Eugene. 'SF, Technoscience, Net.art: The Politics of Extrapolation'. *Art Journal* 59, no. 3 (2000): 64–73.

The 6th Day. [Film] Directed by Roger Spottiswoode. California: Sony Pictures, 2000.

The Island. [Film] Directed by Michael Bay. California: DreamWorks Pictures, 2005.

The Matrix. [Film] Directed by Lana and Lilly Wachowski. Burbank, California: Warner Bros., 1999.

The Pod Generation. [Film] Directed by Sophie Barthes. Belgium: Scope Pictures, 2023.

The X-Files, 'Emily'. [Film] Directed by Kim Manners, written by Vince Gilligan, John Shiban and Frank Spotniz. California: Ten Thirteen Productions, 14 December 1997.

The X-files, 'Essence'. [Film] Directed by Kim Manners, written by Chris Carter. California: Ten Thirteen Productions, 13 May 2001.

Thomasson, Martin. 'A Very Wise Child – Ectogenesis and the Biological Family'. *The Family in the Age of Biotechnology*. Carole Ulanowsky (ed.), 79–89. Suffolk: Ipswich Book Co., 1995.

Thomson, Judith Jarvis. 'A Defense of Abortion'. *Philosophy and Public Affairs* 1, no. 1 (1971): 47–66.

Todorov, Tzvetan. 'Les Catégories du Récit Littéraire [The Categories of Literary Narrative]', Joseph Ketner (trans.). *Papers on Language and Literature* 50, no. 3–4 (2014): 381–424.

Tomita, Taketeru, Atsushi Kaneko, Minoru Toda, Hiromi Morota, Kiyomi Murakumo and KeiichiSato. 'Portable-Sized Artificial Uterine System for Viviparous Shark Embryos'. *MethodsX* 13 (2024): 103063.

Tong, Rosemarie. *Feminist Thought: A Comprehensive Introduction*. Boulder: Westview Press, 1989.

Tranter, Kieran. 'The Speculative Jurisdiction: The Science Fictionality of Law and Technology'. *Griffith Law Review* 20, no. 4 (2011): 817–50.

Tsitas, Evelyn. 'The Role of the Creative Arts in Bioethical Debates'. *Law and Justice Journal* 6, no. 2 (2006): 255–65.

United Nations Educational, Scientific, and Cultural Organization (UNESCO). *Universal Declaration on the Human Genome and Human Rights*. Paris: UNESCO, 1998.

United States Department of Health and Human Services Office of the Inspector General. 'The Emergency Medical Treatment and Labor Act (EMTALA)'. November 2024. Accessed 30 January 2025. https://oig.hhs.gov/reports-and-publications/featured-topics/emtala/

United States Supreme Court. *Roe v. Wade,* 410 U.S. 113 (1973).

Unno, Nobuya, Yoshinori Kuwabara, Takashi Okai, Koichiro Kido, Hirotoshi Nakayama, Akihiko Kikuchi, Yumiko Narumiya, Shiro Kozuma, Yuji Taketani and Masanori Tamura. 'Development of an Artificial Placenta: Survival of Isolated Goat Fetuses for Three Weeks with Umbilical Arteriovenous Extracorporeal Membrane Oxygenation'. *Artificial Organs* 17, no. 12 (1993): 996–1003.

Usada, Haruo, Shimpei Watanabe, Yuichiro Miura, Masatoshi Saito, Gabrielle C. Musk, Judith Rittenscober-Böhm, Hideyuki Ikeda, Shinichi Sato, Takusi Hanita, Tadashi Matsuda, Alan H. Jobe, John P. Newnham, Sarah J. Stock and Matthew W. Kemp. 'Successful Maintenance of Key Physiological Parameters in Preterm Lambs Treated with Ex Vivo Uterine Environment Therapy for a Period of 1 Week'. *American Journal of Obstetrics and Gynecology* 217, no. 4 (2017): 457.

Van Haren, J. S., M. B. van der Hout-van der Jagt, N. Meijer, M. Monincx, F. L. M. Delbressine, X. L. G. Griffith and S. G. Oei. 'Simulation-Based Development: Shaping Clinical Procedures for Extra-uterine Life Support

Technology'. *Advances in Simulation* 8, no. 29 (2023). DOI: 10.1186/s41077-023-00267-y.

Verbeek, Peter-Paul. 'Materializing Morality: Design Ethics and Technological Mediation'. *Science, Technology, & Human Values* 31, no. 3 (2006): 361–80.

Verrips, M., J. S. van Haren, S. G. Oei, A. Moser and M. B. Van der Hout-van der Jagt. 'Clinical Aspects of Umbilical Cord Cannulation During Transfer from the Uterus to a Liquid-Based Perinatal Life Support System for Extremely Premature Infants: A Qualitative Generic Study'. *PLoS One* 18, no. 12 (2023): e0290659.

Verstraten, Peter. *Film Narratology*, Stefan van der Lecq (trans). Toronto: University of Toronto Press, 2009.

Verweij, E. J. (Joanne), and Elselijn Kingma. 'Artificial Placenta – Imminent Ethical Considerations for Research Trials and Clinical Translation'. *American Journal of Bioethics* 23, no. 5 (2023): 85–7.

Vieira, Fátima. 'The Concept of Utopia', in *The Cambridge Companion to Utopian Literature*. Gregory Claeys (ed.), 3–27. Cambridge: Cambridge University Press, 2010.

Vint, Sherryl. 'Introduction: Science Fiction and Biopolitics'. *Science Fiction Film and Television* 4, no. 2 (2011): 161–72.

Wald, Priscilla. 'The Art of Medicine: Cognitive Estrangement, Science Fiction and Medical Ethics'. *The Lancet* 371 (2008): 1908–9.

Walters, William A. W. 'Cloning, Ectogenesis, and Hybrids: Things to Come?' in *Test-Tube Babies: A Guide to Moral Questions, Present Techniques and Future Possibilities*. William A. W. Walters and Peter Singer (eds), 110–18. Melbourne: Oxford University Press, 1982.

Warren, Mary Anne. 'The Moral Significance of Birth'. *Hypatia* 4, no. 3 (1989): 46–65.

Webber, Elizabeth, and Mike Feinsilber. *Merriam-Webster's Dictionary of Allusions*. Massachussetts: Merriam-Webster, 1999.

Weber, David. *At All Costs*. Riverdale, NY: Baen Books, 2005.

Weiner, Jesse, Benjamin Eldon Stevens and Brett M. Rogers. 'Introduction: The Modern Prometheus Turns 200', in *Frankenstein and Its Classics: The Modern Prometheus from Antiquity to Science Fiction*. Jesse Weiner, Benjamin Eldon Stevens and Brett M. Rogers (eds), 1–24. London: Bloomsbury Academic, 2018.

White, Alan R. *The Language of Imagination*. Oxford: Basil Blackwell, 1990.

Wolpert, Lewis. 'The Medawar Lecture 1998: Is Science Dangerous?' *Philosophical Transactions: Biological Sciences* 360, no. 1458 (2005): 1253–8.

Woodward, Kathryn. 'Introduction to Part Three', in *The Gendered Cyborg: A Reader*. Gill Kirkup, Kathryn Woodward and Fiona Hovenden (eds), 161–9. London: Routledge, 2000.

World Health Organization. 'Managing Complications in Pregnancy and Childbirth: A Guide for Midwives and Doctors – Second Edition'. February 2017. Accessed 29 January 2025. https://www.who.int/publications/i/item/9789241565493

Yoo, Jihun. 'Transhumanist Impulse, Utopian Vision, and Reversing Dystopia in Margaret Atwood's *Oryx and Crake* and Octavia E. Butler's *Dawn*'. *The Modern Language Review* 114, no. 4 (2019): 662–81.

Zachary, G. Pascal. 'Ethics for a Very Small World'. *Foreign Policy* 137 (2003): 108–9.

Zaki, Hoda M. 'Utopia, Dystopia, and Ideology in the Science Fiction of Octavia Butler (Utopie, dystopie et idéologie dans la science-fiction d'Octavia Butler)'. *Science Fiction Studies* 17, no. 2 (1990): 239–51.

Zamyatin, Yevgeny. *We*. New York: Modern Library, 2006.

Zaremberg, Gisela, Constanza Tabbush and Elisabeth Jay Friedman. 'Feminism(s) and Anti-gender Backlash: Lessons from Latin America'. *International Feminist Journal of Politics* 23, no. 4 (2021): 527–34.

Zimmerman, Jan. 'Technology and the Future of Women: Haven't We Met Somewhere Before?' *Women's Studies International Forum* 4, no. 3 (1981): 355–67.

Index

abortion 2, 15, 20, 49, 85, 97, 126
opposition 15, 20, 49, 158
rights and access 21, 23, 25, 32–7, 148, 155
in science fiction 41, 48, 143
Adami, Valentina 68
adoption 15, 22, 34, 36, 111–12
in science fiction 77
afrofuturism 42, 141–2
Agar, Nicholas 100
amniotic fluid
in science fiction 51, 53
synthetic 16–17
anticipatory ethics 42, 199, 153–6
See also, Speculative bioethics
artificial amniotic and placental technologies (AAPT) 31
See also, ectogenesis
artificial placenta 16–17, 27, 41, 148
See also, ectogenesis
artificial womb
See, ectogenesis
Asimov, Isaac
The Dying Night 61–2
Atwood, Margaret
Oryx and Crake 135
autonomy 10, 21, 48, 67, 120
reproductive 2, 20–1, 23, 30, 33, 35–7, 39, 41, 130
in science fiction 77, 84, 92, 114

Batman 85–7
Baylis, Françoise 111
Bayne, Tim 42, 75
See also, Kolers, Avery
Berkeley, George 46
bio-bag 5, 16–17, 23
in science fiction 84, 149
bioengineered wombs 3, 42
bioethics
creative utopian 160
definitions 42, 45, 65–8, 93–5
education 55, 57, 109–110, 112–17, 119–21, 126, 131
history and development 7–11, 23–5
-in-literature 6–7, 68, 112, 119–24, 126, 143
biopolitics 11, 93–95, 104, 107, 109, 111–12, 116–17
birth
See, childbirth
See, pregnancy
Bostrom, Nick 52
Bould, Mark 61
Braidotti, Rosi 86–7
Brave New World
See, Huxley, Aldous
Brecht, Bertolt
V-Effekt 60–1
See also, estrangement
Brittain, Vera
Halcyon 88–89
Browne, Tamara Kayali 28–9, 38
Bujold, Lois McMaster
Ethan of Athos 82–3
Shards of Honor 41
Vorkosigan saga 41, 115
Butler, Octavia E.
Dawn 119, 126, 133–48, 152
Xenogenesis trilogy 42

Cannold, Leslie 15, 34, 158
Carroll, Noël 57, 74
Cartwright, Lisa 55, 112
See also, Moral
Cavaliere, Giulia 159
Chambers, Tod 66–7, 108–9
characterization 55–57, 66–8, 71, 90, 108, 110, 114, 121, 124, 127–9, 131, 142
See also, narratology
childbirth 2
caesarean 28–30, 36
health risks 3, 8, 19, 29, 39, 71, 77

legal and social definitions 8, 29, 31–3, 35, 37, 75, 130, 154
in science fiction 51–3, 56, 76–7, 79, 82, 88–90, 139, 141–3, 146, 149
See also, pregnancy
Children's Hospital of Philadelphia 16
Childress, James F. 67
Choi, Julie 144
cloning 12–13, 69, 79–80, 97–8, 103, 105, 108, 110, 114
Dolly the sheep 98–99
in science fiction 51–2, 54, 63, 69–71, 73, 80–2, 92, 94, 101–2, 113, 117, 125, 134, 140
clustered regularly interspaced short palindromic repeats (CRISPR) 85, 105
Cohen, Glenn 85, 98
Coma 122
commodification 51, 79, 90, 114
Corea, Gena 8, 43, 83
Cowart, Dax 48, 67, 126
Csicsery-Ronay Jr, Istvan 47–8, 115–16

Davis, Dena S. 102
De Bie, Felix 17, 24–8, 30–2, 35–6, 38, 40, 42
De Beauvoir, Simone 19
defamiliarization effect 42
See also, estrangement
Delany, Samuel R. 58, 127
Descartes, Rene 46
designer babies 76, 102, 106
See also, genetic engineering
design ethics 18, 119, 147–53
Dutch design week 152
Dick, Philip K. 58
dignity 78–81, 105, 114
Doctor Who 62–3
Duden, Barbara 49, 130
Dworkin, Andrea 8
dystopia 23, 66, 80–1, 98–9, 101–2, 106–7, 113–16, 125, 135, 155, 157–8
definitions 12, 64, 91, 94, 97
feminist 13, 95, 135–6, 143–4

ectogenesis
animal trials 7, 16, 18, 26, 96, 134
arguments in favour 1–3, 5–7, 9, 11–12, 18–20, 38, 77, 111, 114, 144, 157
attitudes towards 1, 3, 15, 38, 96–7, 157–8
Catholic perspectives 28
history and development 1, 7, 15–18, 22, 96
Islamic perspectives 28
in science fiction 12, 22–3, 40, 54, 91–2, 94, 101, 113, 115–16, 139–41
selection for 25–8
terminology 30–2, 163
ectogestation
See, ectogenesis
Edwards, Robert 22, 69–70, 72, 74
See also, Steptoe, Patrick
Eindhoven University of Technology 17, 152
equality
sexual 1, 5–7, 11–13, 18–19, 82, 87–91, 114, 128, 157
in science fiction 116, 128, 155
See also, inequality
estrangement 42, 60–2, 91–2, 157–8
See also, defamiliarization effect
eugenics 77, 84, 100, 106–7
See also, Agar, Nicholas
eutopia
See, utopia
extra-uterine environment for newborn development (EXTEND) 16, 23, 32, 40
See also, ectogenesis
extra-uterine foetal incubation (EUFI) 96
See also, ectogenesis
ex-utero gestation 31, 35
See also, ectogenesis
ex-vivo gestation
See, ectogenesis
ex-vivo uterine environment (EVE) 16
See also, ectogenesis

fabula 127–8
Farquhar, Dion 5, 9, 50, 86, 88, 155
feminism 13, 19, 143
fundamentalist 9, 11, 82, 87
liberal 10–11, 64–5, 119, 126, 137, 144
Marxist 65
radical 7–8, 155

Ferreira, Aline, 91–2
Firestone, Shulamith 11, 87, 89–90
The Dialectic of Sex 7–8, 89
focalization 70–1, 88, 126–33, 142–7
See also, narratology
foetus
experimentation 23, 26–7, 97
health risks 2–3, 17, 20, 77, 86
premature 17, 27
rights 30–2, 39, 50, 131
terminology
foetonate 24, 30–2, 36, 41
gestateling 30, 32, 41
Foucault, Michel 95, 131
Frankenstein
character 22, 70, 73, 94–5, 99, 104–5, 109–10
See also, Shelley, Mary
Freedman, Carl 61–2
free indirect discourse
See, narratology
Fringe 78
Frye, Northrop 55
fuzzy set 59

Gattaca 94–5, 100, 103, 105–7, 111, 114–15
gay
See, LGBTI
genetic engineering 13, 74, 97, 106
of crops 103
in science fiction 76–8, 84–5, 94–5, 102–4, 106–8, 111, 116–17, 136–7, 140–4
See also, clustered regularly interspaced short palindromic repeats (CRISPR)
See also, hybrids
Genette, Gérard 129, 133
Ghost in the Shell 123
Gilman, Charlotte Perkins
Herland 64
Green, Ronald M. 100, 102

Haldane, J. B. S. 22, 51–2, 106, 113
Hamilton, Sheryl N. 48, 98, 101, 110, 116
Haraway, Donna 5
Hobbes, Thomas 46
Horn, Claire 7–8
Hughes, James J. 112–13
human farms 8, 23, 73, 78–9, 81, 134
See also, *The Matrix*
Hume, David 46
humidicribs
See, incubators
Huxley, Aldous
Brave New World 23, 55, 72, 80–2, 91, 94–7, 100–2, 107–8, 113–16, 125
hybrids
animal-human 73–5, 84–5, 134
human-alien 75, 133–5, 137, 139, 141, 144
See also, clustered regularly interspaced short palindromic repeats (CRISPR)
See also, genetic engineering

imagination 4, 6, 39–40, 42, 48, 50, 55, 66, 86, 93, 99, 117, 124, 149, 157, 160
theories of 45–8
Immega, Guy
Super-Earth Mother 83–4, 149–50
incubators 3, 17, 22, 24, 32, 35, 37, 47
Side shows 22
inequality
financial 10, 20, 23, 25, 54
political and social 20, 54, 107, 159
racial 9–10, 38, 90, 137, 143
sexual 4–5, 11, 15, 18–21, 29, 87–91, 114, 116, 134, 142, 144, 155, 157, 159
See also, equality
infertility 2–3, 19, 39, 84, 111, 159, 163
in science fiction 134
social 2, 83–4, 154, 159, 163
informed consent 10, 26, 29, 34, 36, 85, 133, 136, 144, 147
Inhorn, Marcia C. 28
in vitro fertilization (IVF) 7, 22, 36, 71, 85, 111, 113, 154
history and development 7, 69–71, 97, 113, 159
Islamic perspectives 28
opposition 9, 22, 72, 74, 97, 112, 159
in science fiction 115

James, Henry 129
Jameson, Fredric 60, 115–16

Jasanoff, Sheila 55–6
Junior 151

Kant, Immanuel 47, 79
Kass, Leon 53, 72, 100–1
Kendal, Evie 3, 5, 9, 28–9, 38, 84, 93, 144, 148, 159
Kingma, Elselijn 26, 29, 31
Kirby, David A. 105–6, 116
Kitzinger, Jenny 102–3
Kolers, Avery 42, 75
  See also, Bayne, Tim
Kristeva, Julia 54
Kyle XY 76–8

Lanphier, Elizabeth 42, 199
  See also, Lomotey-Nakon, Leah
Lanser, Susan S. 132–3
Lantos, John D. 26, 43, 106, 112–13
Latimer, Heather 110, 154
Lauritzen, Paul 46, 48, 50, 53
Le Guin, Ursula K. 6, 153
  The Dispossessed 64
  The Left Hand of Darkness 116, 155, 157
LGBTI 3, 12, 21, 38–9, 89, 108, 154
Livingston, Dennis 5–6
Lomotey-Nakon, Leah 42, 119
  See also, Lanphier, Elizabeth

mad scientist 69–73, 103–4, 133
Marxism 60, 62, 65
Mercurio, Mark 26–7, 32, 40
Meyers, Diana 4
Miéville, China 61
Milner, Andrew 59, 65, 81
moral
  emotions 45, 66, 68, 130, 142, 155
  spectatorship 55, 66, 111–12, 156
More, Thomas
  Utopia 58
Moylan, Tom 64
Murphy, Julien 7

narratology 6, 45, 57, 126–31, 155
  feminist 131–3
    See also, Lanser, Susan S.
  film 128–9
  voice 67, 144
    free indirect discourse 144–7
  See also, fabula
Nelson, Hilde Lindemann 65–6, 119, 124–6, 128, 131–2
Nineteen Eighty-Four
  See, Orwell, George
novum 60, 62–3, 76, 91, 116, 137
Nussbaum, Martha 65–6

O'Brien, Mary, 19, 21, 86–7
Orwell, George
  Nineteen Eighty-Four 97

Partridge, Emily A. 16, 23
patriarchy 5, 8–9, 19, 43, 64, 82–3, 135–7
Piercy, Marge
  Woman on the Edge of Time 64, 76, 87–90, 114, 116, 157–8
point of view 70, 115, 124, 126, 128–32, 142, 144, 147
  See also, focalization
pregnancy
  economic burdens 3–4, 18–19, 33, 155
  ectopic 41
  legal risks 10–11, 19–21, 29–30, 86, 158
  over-medicalization 8, 38, 40–1, 131, 143
  risks to health 2–4, 10, 12, 19, 21, 25, 29, 39, 126
pre-implantation genetic diagnosis (PGD) 77
premature 2–3, 17, 22, 24, 26–7, 32, 37, 148
  See also, foetus
procreative beneficence 77
  See also, Savulescu, Julian
Prince, Gerald 126–7
pronatalism 1, 4–5, 144

queer
  See, LGBTI

Räsänen, Joona 34–5
Raymond, Janice G. 19–20, 87
robotics 100, 122–3, 136
Romanis, Chloe Elizabeth 29, 30–2, 148, 153, 160
Rothman, Barbara Katz 8
Rowland, Robyn 8–9

Russ, Joanna
The Female Man 64

same sex
See, LGBTI
Sargent, Lyman Tower 116–17
Sartre, Jean-Paul 47
saviour sibling 71
Savulescu, Julian 77
Schiavo, Terri 48, 126
Schuelke, Gertrude 145
science fiction
genre definition 57–65
role in science communication 11, 95–100, 107–11, 123
Sedgwick, Helen
The Growing Season 43, 90
Segers, Seppe 24, 28–9, 34, 158
sexual violence 35, 155
in science fiction 74, 136–8, 140, 142, 144
Shelley, Mary
Frankenstein 54, 58, 69, 72, 94–5, 100, 102–5, 107–8, 115
Silver, Lee M. 91, 98–9, 107, 111
Singer, Peter 9, 26
slippery slope 71–2, 103, 154
Smajdor, Anna 4, 10, 159
sonogram
See, ultrasound
Space: Above and Beyond 40, 76
space colonization 83–5, 134, 136
See also, Immega, Guy
speculative bioethics 45, 97, 102, 109, 115, 152–4
See also, anticipatory ethics
See also, design ethics
Spencer, Kathleen L. 62
Splice 73–5, 104
Squier, Susan M. 11, 49, 88, 110
Star Trek 76, 112, 121
The Next Generation 100
Voyager 41
Steiger, Eric, 33, 37, 75, 87
Steptoe, Patrick 22, 70
Sudenkaarne, Tiia 28–9, 38
Superboy 86
Super-Earth Mother
See, Immega, Guy
surrogacy 2, 21–2, 28, 36, 71, 112, 134
in science fiction 52
Suvin, Darko 59–65, 76, 91, 110, 137, 160–1
See also, novum

termination of pregnancy
See, abortion
The Boys from Brazil 110
The Island 23, 50–6, 63, 70–1, 73, 78, 88, 104, 149
The Matrix 23, 50, 53, 55, 78–9, 96, 104, 149
The Pod Generation 23, 89–91, 150–2, 155
therapeutic misconception 26, 29
The Silent Scream 48–50
The 6th Day 70, 73, 88
The Terminator 82–3
The X-Files 75–6
transgender health 3, 163
See also, LGBTI
transplant 105, 122–3
in science fiction 71
uterine 3
xenotransplantation 75
Tranter, Kieran 71, 93, 97, 102

ultrasound 49
images 50, 130, 150
in science fiction 149
Universal Declaration on the Human Genome and Human Rights 80
utopia
definitions 116, 125, 161
feminist 12, 64, 68, 88–9, 114, 137, 144, 157–9
See also, dystopia

Verweij, E. J. 26, 29, 31
Vint, Sheryl 11, 94, 109
visual bioethics 45–6, 48–51, 53, 128, 148, 155
See also, Lauritzen, Paul

Wells, Deane 9, 26
Williams, Raymond 59

Wittgenstein, Ludwig 47, 59
Wolfe, Gary K. 58
Woman on the Edge of Time
  See, Piercy, Marge
women's empowerment 5, 11, 19, 23,
    64, 136

X-man 85–6

yuck factor 13, 45, 51–5, 149

Zamyatin, Yevgeny
  We 77

www.ingramcontent.com/pod-product-compliance
Ingram Content Group UK Ltd.
Pitfield, Milton Keynes, MK11 3LW, UK
UKHW020809290926
15470UKWH00003B/1047

9 781350 542976